The Low Vision Handbook

The Low Vision Handbook

Barbara Brown, CO, COMT, MEd
Eye Care Specialists, P.C.
Norwood, Massachusetts

‖‖ The Basic Bookshelf for Eyecare Professionals

Series Editors: Janice K. Ledford • Ken Daniels • Robert Campbell

SLACK Incorporated, 6900 Grove Road, Thorofare, NJ 08086-9447

Publisher: John H. Bond
Editorial Director: Amy E. Drummond
Creative Director: Linda Baker
Assistant Editor: Miriam Priest

Brown, Barbara
The low vision handbook/Barbara Brown.
p. cm.—(The basic bookshelf for eyecare professionals; 3)
Includes bibliographical references and index.
ISBN 1-55642-329-2 (alk. paper)
1. Low vision—Handbooks, manuals, etc. I Title. II. Series.
[DNLM: 1. Vision, Subnormal. WW 140 B877L 1997]
RE91.B75 1997
617.7'12—dc21
DNLM/DLC   97-10169
for Library of Congress   CIP

Printed in the United States of America

Published by: SLACK Incorporated
               6900 Grove Road
               Thorofare, NJ 08086-9447 USA
               Telephone: 609-848-1000
               Fax: 609-853-5991

Contact SLACK Incorporated for more information about other books in this field or about the availability of our books from distributors outside the United States.

Last digit is print number: 10 9 8 7 6 5 4 3 2 1

Dedication

For my mother Beverly Anne Childs, and my father Donald Arthur Brown.

Contents

Dedication . . . . *v*

Acknowledgments . . . . *ix*

About the Author . . . . *xi*

The Study Icons . . . . *xiii*

Chapter 1. Introduction to Low Vision 1

Chapter 2. Optical Low Vision Aids 7

Chapter 3. Nonoptical and Electronic Low Vision Aids 29

Chapter 4. History Taking 45

Chapter 5. Assessment of Visual Function .57

Chapter 6. Selecting Aids for Individuals 67

Chapter 7. Rehabilitation and Referrals 77

Chapter 8. Setting Up a Low Vision Service 89

Chapter 9. The Psychology of Visual Loss .97

Chapter 10. Case Histories 109

Appendix I: A Glossary of Basic Optical Terms 123

Appendix II: Internet Addresses of Low Vision Resources 129

Index 133

Acknowledgments

This book is the result of 18 years of work in visual rehabilitation, low vision, and ophthalmic technology. It could not have been written without the expert early guidance and support of Purvis Ponder and Eileen Reed of Florida State University, Barbara Cassin of the University of Florida, and Malcolm Luxenburg of the Medical College of Georgia. I thank each of them for unselfishly sharing their knowledge and experience, and for nurturing my interest in low vision care.

I would also like to thank the many people who provided current information on all the topics in this book. Janet Hession and Sandy Daly from the Massachusetts Commission for the Blind, and Susan Laventure from the Perkins School for the Blind were especially helpful. Dina Rosenbaum and Robert McGillivray of the Carroll Center for the Blind CABLE technology program devoted a large amount of their valuable time explaining the latest in electronic devices and computer assistive technology. Frank Lazenby and Deborah Hudson provided their photographic expertise. Jan Ledford has been a superb editor, offering just the right amount of encouragement and advice. Most importantly, Ann Stewart of the Center for the Visually Impaired in Atlanta devoted a great deal of time and dedication providing excellent suggestions, photographs, and friendship.

My husband, Harry Castleman, has been willing to share humor, encouragement, and valuable computer time while we both had concurrent publication deadlines. My delightful daughter, Claire Castleman, has given me reason to procrastinate and reason to achieve.

About the Author

Barbara Brown holds a degree in Visual Disabilities and certifications in Ophthalmic Medical Technology and Orthoptics. She has provided low vision care to patients since 1980 in low vision clinics and private ophthalmology practices in Georgia, Florida, and Massachusetts. She has published several journal articles on low vision care, and was involved in the development of the low vision section for the JCAHPO® certification examinations. She currently works and resides in Canton, Massachusetts.

The Study Icons

The *Basic Bookshelf For Eyecare Professionals* is quality educational material designed for professionals in all branches of eyecare. Because so many of you want to expand your careers, we have made a special effort to include information needed for certification exams. When these study icons appear in the margin of a *Series* book, it is your cue that the material next to the icon is listed as a criteria item for a certification examination. Please use this key to identify the appropriate icon:

OptA	optometric assistant
OptT	optometric technician
OphA	ophthalmic assistant
OphT	ophthalmic technician
OphMT	ophthalmic medical technologist
LV	low vision subspecialty[*]
Srg	ophthalmic surgical assisting subspecialty
CL	contact lens registry
Optn	opticianry
RA	retinal angiographer
OPRA	ophthalmic photographer and retinal angiographer

[*]Note: Because this icon applies to the entire book, it will not appear anywhere on the pages.

Chapter 1

Introduction to Low Vision

- Low vision is not defined by specific acuity limits. It includes any functional visual loss after the correction of refractive error and presbyopia.

- Low vision aids are defined as devices that improve the efficiency of remaining vision.

- Complete low vision care includes rehabilitation as well as optical aids.

- Assistants are extremely valuable in providing low vision care.

History of Low Vision Care

The term "low vision" was coined in the second half of the 20th century. Prior to that time, the majority of people in medical and rehabilitation communities paid little heed to the issue. They dealt with visual impairment in black and white terms; a patient was either sighted or blind. Blind patients were taught Braille and sent to schools for the blind. If any of them had residual vision, its use was discouraged in order to "save" the sight. The theory was that by using the eyes, they could be damaged further. These "sight saving" techniques were widely accepted practice from 1913 until 1950.

Although small efforts were being made in various settings to help those who were "partially blind," it took a world war to make substantial changes. After World War II, many military men had service-related disabilities. Enabling veterans to return to the work force despite a "partial disability" was the major thrust behind the growth of the field of low vision. The first low vision aids were fit in 1953. Our understanding of the needs specific to low vision patients has continued to improve, and in the 1990s low vision services finally have been recognized as a significant part of patient treatment.

Low vision has many definitions, but in general it is any loss of *functional vision* that persists *after* the correction of distance refractive error and common age-related or surgical presbyopia. This definition varies according to the needs of each individual patient. For instance, a patient with 20/60 best corrected visual acuity (BVA) may have a severe functional impairment. Consider Mr. Johnson who is a taxi driver and can no longer pass his driver's license renewal exam. He needs low vision assistance to maintain his profession, income, dignity, and independence. By contrast, Mrs. Thomas, an elderly woman with 20/200 BVA, may need little or no optical intervention if she is illiterate and does not drive or work. She may do very well with her daily tasks. In just a few home visits, rehabilitation personnel may teach her organizational skills to locate desired objects more easily. She can also be taught skills to help her maneuver in the local neighborhood. With a supportive family, this may be all the rehabilitation needed in spite of a severe visual loss. Because of these unique individual differences, the interpretation of a patient's needs becomes the challenge of low vision care.

Other terms are used interchangeably with low vision. Examples of these are "visually impaired," "partially sighted," "partially blind," "visually challenged," and "subnormal vision." Sometimes the term indicates or implies the level of visual loss such as "severely visually impaired" and "legally blind." Legal blindness is the only one of these terms that has a specific legal definition. Legal blindness is defined as BVA of 20/200 or less in the better seeing eye, or a visual field loss such that the maximum diameter of the visual field is 20° or less (even if the measurable acuity is good). Therefore, all people who are legally blind also have low vision, but not all low vision patients are legally blind. Be careful not to interchange these terms casually. They have different implications for the patient in terms of availability of social services and tax advantages.

"Visual efficiency" refers to an individual's functional visual ability in spite of loss. Using acuity as a cutoff for vision services does not take into account the fact that visual efficiency varies greatly among individuals. Two people with the same diagnosis and the same level of measurable acuity may meet their visual tasks in very different ways. The acuity level may be devastating to one person and restrict his or her entire lifestyle. To another person it may be more of an inconvenience than a hardship, and he or she will develop creative ways of adapting to various situations. The use of low vision aids increases visual efficiency. Visual efficiency also depends on training, experience, intelligence level, and personality characteristics of the individual, as well as other disabilities that may interfere with normal function.

OphMT

OptT

OptA

What the Patient Needs to Know

- Legal blindness is a specific term that implies one of the following:

  a. Your "best" eye cannot see any better than 20/200 while you are wearing the best correcting lens available in your glasses. (This does not mean your vision with low vision aids.)

  b. The diameter of your side vision is very small—20° or less—regardless of how well you see small objects.

- Poor vision that is correctable by glasses or is better than either of these two definitions does not qualify you for federal or state services for the blind.

Providing Low Vision Services

A good low vision clinic does more than prescribe optical devices. It meets the challenges of various types of visual loss by joining with rehabilitation personnel to offer a "total package" to patients. This package consists of many parts, and if any of them are neglected the patient is not served fully. These elements include training in the use of optical aids, recommendations for nonoptical devices, occupational and educational help, orientation and mobility training, and assistance with the tasks of daily living. Counselling help with the emotional and psychological aspects of adjusting to loss of vision are also paramount for both the patient and family members.

Because all of these needs must be addressed, many private practitioners shy away from offering low vision services. They may refer all patients to established low vision clinics or social service agencies and hope their needs are met there. Worst of all, they may ignore the issue altogether. None of these options is ideal. Referral to a full-service low vision clinic is the best of these choices, but has its own limitations, including the lack of these clinics in nonmetropolitan areas. Sometimes a "low vision clinic" is simply an office that will order optical aids. The rehabilitation needs of the patient may still be overlooked. Also, in this case the low vision care will be provided by someone who has no history or rapport with the patient.

Private practitioners who want to provide good low vision services should be prepared to do the following:

1. Provide low vision optical evaluations themselves and make referrals to agencies that provide rehabilitation services.
2. If a practitioner refers the patient to a low vision clinic instead, the practitioner should ascertain in advance if that clinic works closely with rehabilitation personnel. If it does not, the practitioner should be responsible for making a second referral to an agency that does provide that service.
3. Discuss the issue of visual loss tactfully with the patient, honestly answering all questions about the medical diagnosis and prognosis so the patient does not hold on to false hopes or unrealistic fears.
4. Refer the patient and family members to counselling services to deal with the loss of vision and its accompanying loss of independence.
5. Provide regular follow-up low vision care to ascertain if there are any further needs that are not being met, in addition to addressing medical issues.

The Role of the Low Vision Assistant

The optometric or ophthalmic assistant has an important role in this process. As a low vision assistant he or she will be responsible for coordinating referrals to the many social service agencies that provide help with adjustment to visual loss. Also, because the assistant usually spends the most time taking the patient's history and discussing personal issues, a thorough knowledge of the needs of visually impaired patients is paramount in order to ask the right questions. By understanding the complete needs of each low vision patient, assistants can act as advocates in the process of obtaining care. Follow-up care and training in the use of optical aids is of vital importance in the patient's success, and these are also skills that can be provided by the low vision assistant.

It is the intent of this book to make each step in the low vision process clear for the assistant who is going to provide the most complete care. The assistant who only needs to understand which agencies are helpful to individual patients and where to find those agencies in your area will also find this book invaluable. These responsibilities sound complicated, but with very little effort it is possible for every ophthalmology or optometry office to ensure that their patients with low vision receive this full range of services. Very few low vision aids are complicated, and many social service agencies are already present in most areas to meet the needs of your patients. It is simply a matter of locating the services and understanding how to make referrals. Then the process becomes easy as well as rewarding.

In the following chapters, you will learn what you need to know to begin a low vision service in your office. Optics knowledge required for low vision care is provided first. You will also be introduced to proper and complete low vision history taking that includes social as well as medical concerns. By asking the appropriate questions in the beginning, you will know what type of low vision aids to try and when the patient may need referrals for social services. Techniques to test visual acuity and refractive error of low vision patients will also be presented. Many routine tests must be modified for patients with subnormal vision, but very little is needed in the way of specialized equipment. Optical and nonoptical low vision aids, as well as electronic devices, will be discussed in detail.

Rehabilitation services important to patients with a visual disability will be explained. Suggestions for referrals will be given, along with addresses for specific agencies and vendors. This is neither an exhaustive nor scholarly work on low vision care, but it should allow assistants at any level to begin offering care to low vision patients in any setting.

Chapter 2

Optical Low Vision Aids

KEY POINTS

- Optical low vision aids use magnification to enlarge retinal image size.

- Spectacles require an eye-to-print distance equal to the focal length of the lens.

- Hand magnifiers require a lens-to-print distance equal to the focal length of the lens. Distance correction should be worn when using hand magnifiers.

- Stand magnifiers require either reading correction or sufficient accommodative ability.

- Telescopes can be used by children, adults, and patients with nystagmus or visual field loss. They are the only low vision aid used at distance.

Any professional or assistant who is dealing with low vision must have a knowledge of the basic optics involved in magnification. For the reader with little optical background, this overview presents the most important subjects in relatively simple terms. The dictionary of optical terms in the Appendix may be used as a supplement.

Magnification

The purpose of low vision aids is to magnify the retinal image of an object. By enlarging the size of the image that is projected onto the retinal surface, it is more likely that the image will be seen by the remaining healthy tissue surrounding compromised areas. For example, if a macular scotoma is 4° in size, it would be very difficult to see a letter that subtends a 4° angle. Every time the patient tried to view the image it would fall on the scotoma and disappear (Figure 2-1). If the same retinal image is doubled in size it will then subtend an 8° angle on the retina. The same central scotoma will diminish the clarity of the image, but not eliminate it. This enlarging of retinal images is the primary goal of all optical low vision aids.

There are four types of magnification used to achieve enlargement of retinal images:

1. Relative Size Magnification

   The object actually is made larger. Examples include large-print books and enlarged numbers on telephone dial pads. There is a direct relationship of increased object size to increased retinal image size. By just doubling the size of the actual object, the retinal image size will also be doubled and easier to see. No change in optical correction is necessary except to provide clarity.

2. Relative Distance Magnification

   As objects are brought closer to the eye, the retinal image size is again enlarged proportionally. A closer object takes up a larger portion of the visual field and the image will be larger on the retina. As the distance changes, the retinal image size also changes, or is "magnified," relative to that change in distance. It is still necessary to focus the image by means of lenses or accommodation.

3. Angular Magnification

   Angular magnification is a complicated type of magnification that occurs from a system of lenses such as are found in telescopes and binoculars. Divergent light rays leaving the system cause images to appear to be coming from a closer distance than the actual location of the object. The image we see is a virtual image. Our brain is aware that objects appear smaller as they get further away, so when distant objects appear larger, our brain interprets them as being closer.

4. Projection Magnification

   Print or images may be enlarged by projection, (eg, when the image on a small piece of 35-mm film is enlarged by means of a slide projector). Movie film projected to fill a movie screen and acetate sheets enlarged by an overhead projector are other examples. In low vision, closed circuit televisions (CCTVs) use this type of magnification very successfully.

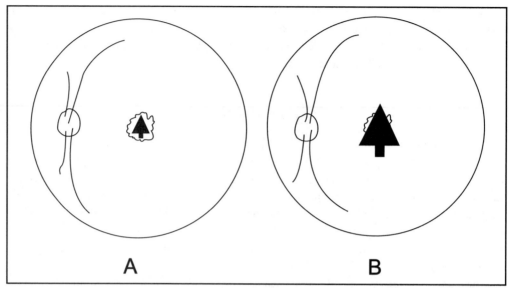

Figure 2-1. If the retinal image is the same size as a central scotoma it cannot be seen (A). If the image is doubled in size (B), enough of it can be seen to interpret the image.

Diopters and Focal Distance

Knowledge of two optical principles, diopters (D) and focal distance, are vital to understanding the optics of all low vision aids.

Diopters

The power of a lens is measured in diopters. A diopter is defined as the optical power needed to focus parallel rays of light at 1 meter. In practical terms for low vision, to focus the image of an object held at 1 meter, a 1-D lens is needed.

As the distance is shortened, the power needed to focus an image increases in inverse proportion. Cutting the image distance in half doubles the dioptric demand. For example, at ½ m there is a 2 D power requirement (1/2 m = 2/1 D). At 1/3 m, 3 diopters are needed (1/3 m = 3/1 D), and so on (Table 2-1). This standard principle is used when prescribing reading adds for patients with presbyopia as well as in low vision.

To calculate the power of a lens needed to focus at a particular distance, first convert that distance into centimeters, then divide into 100 cm. The result is the dioptric power. Suppose an object is at ½ m. Converted to centimeters, the object is 50 cm away. Divide 100 by 50 and the result is 2 D of power needed to focus at this distance. The formula to remember is D = 100/F, where D is diopters and F is the focal length (or distance).

Focal Length

Focal length is the distance at which a lens focuses parallel rays of light. To determine focal length, divide 1 m (100 cm) by the dioptric power of the lens (Figure 2-2). As you can see, this is the opposite or inverse of the diopter formula. For example, a 5-D lens has a focal length of 20 cm (100 cm ÷ 5 D = 20 cm). In general terms, focal length refers to the distance at which a lens will make an image appear to be in focus. For example, using the above situation, the 5-D lens

Table 2-1
Diopter/Distance Chart

Distance to the Object	Power Needed to Focus Image
5 cm (1/20 m)	20 D
10 cm (1/10 m)	10 D
12.5 cm (1/8 m)	8 D
20 cm (1/5 m)	5 D
25 cm (1/4 m)	4 D
33.3 cm (1/3 m)	3 D
40 cm (1/2.5 m)	2.5 D
100 cm (1 m)	1 D
200 cm (2 m)	0.5 D

D = diopters.

will focus an object that is 20 cm away, but will not focus one that is 10 cm or 30 cm away. The formula for focal length is $F = 100/D$, where F is the focal length and D is diopters of power in the lens.

"×" Notation

An object of a given size "projects" an image on the retina of the viewing eye. This retinal image is also of a given size, usually measured in seconds, minutes, or degrees of arc. When discussing magnification, "×" refers to the number of times the retinal image is enlarged in size. 1× means there is no change in the size, 2× means the image is twice the "normal" size, 3× means the image is three times the normal size, etc. This notation can be confusing because it depends on what is being used as a reference. Is a 2× image twice as large as one from an object viewed at 1 m, or twice as large as one from an object viewed at 10 cm?

For common low vision notation, 40 cm is considered to be the standard reference distance. That means that a 1× magnifier has the power needed to focus (not enlarge) an image at 40 cm. In diopters, the power necessary to focus at 40 centimeters is +2.50. A 1× lens, then, is equivalent in power to +2.50 diopters.

The power of a lens that can make an image appear to be twice its size is 2×. If an image is 1× at 40 cm, it would have to be moved to 20 cm (half the distance) to be viewed as twice the size. The power needed to focus at 20 cm is +5.00 D. A 2× magnifier, then, is equivalent to a 5-D lens with a focal distance of 20 cm. A 4× magnifier is the same as a 10-D lens with a focal distance of 10 cm, etc. (Table 2-2).

Some manufacturers use 25 cm instead of 40 cm as their reference distance for labelling lenses. In that case, 1× would represent a lens that would focus at 25 cm, or a +4.00-D lens. A 2× magnifier would represent an +8.00 lens.

Be careful because it is possible to order a 2× lens for a patient based on satisfactory performance in the office; but when the magnifier arrives the patient may not be able to read with it. Perhaps the one you tried in the office was an +8.00 lens and the one that arrived was a +5.00 lens, although they are both labelled 2×. To avoid this problem, read all magnifiers on a lensometer as they arrive in your office. Each low vision aid should be labelled according to dioptric power rather than in terms of × so the notation is standardized in your office.

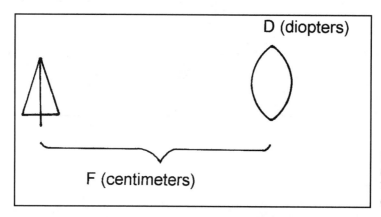

Figure 2-2. To calculate diopters, divide 100 by F. To calculate focal length, divide 100 by D.

Table 2-2
Magnification Power Equivalencies

Magnification (×)	Dioptric Equivalent (40 cm Reference)	Dioptric Equivalent (25 cm Reference)
1	+2.50	+4.00
2	+5.00	+8.00
3	+7.50	+12.00
4	+10.00	+16.00
5	+12.50	+20.00
6	+15.00	+24.00
10	+25.00	+40.00

Optical Low Vision Aids

There is nothing magic about optical low vision aids. They are simply magnifying lenses of various powers, sizes, and styles. They include spectacles, hand magnifiers, stand magnifiers, and loupes. Some of them have been altered from their basic style to meet the specific needs of low vision patients, but most are standard styles that are available to the general public.

Spectacles

Spectacles are the low vision aids that are most often prescribed, and are the aid of choice in most situations (Figure 2-3). They are simply reading glasses with higher powers than normal. These higher powers provide a shorter focal distance, resulting in relative distance magnification. Low vision spectacles can range in power from 4 D to 64 D. For clear focus, the reading distance should be equal to the focal length of the lenses. In a 4-D lens the reading distance would be 25 cm. In a pair of 64 D reading spectacles, the focal distance would be 1.6 cm from the eye. Stronger powers than 64 D in spectacles alone would render the reading distance closer than is humanly possible. The most common powers are 4 D to 16 D.

When selecting spectacles for a patient, it is important to keep in mind the patient's refractive error. If a patient is 4 D myopic, he already has a "built-in" 4 D reading add. If the dioptric demand for appropriate magnification is 6 D, only the remaining 2 D needs to be provided in spectacles. The "internal" 4 D from the myopia makes up the difference. This still represents a 6

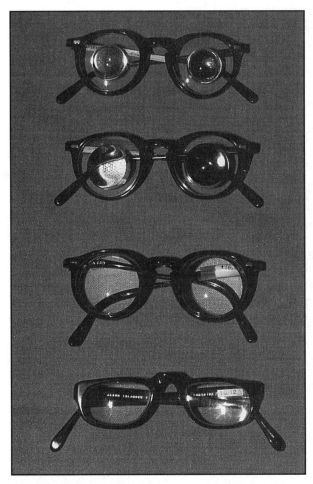

Figure 2-3. Low vision spectacles.

D reading *add* for this patient, and the reading distance remains 16.7 cm (100 ÷ 6 = 16.7). Do not be misled because the actual power of the glasses is only 2 D.

Similarly, a patient with hyperopia must have enough plus to correct their hypermetropia as well as the necessary reading add. For instance, a patient with 3 D of hyperopia who requires a 10 D reading add will need +13.00 spectacles for reading. This provides the 3 D needed for emmetropia, added to the 10 D needed for the near focus.

Also include any significant astigmatic correction in either case. "Significant correction" refers to any cylinder power that makes the image subjectively clearer to the patient. If no subjective improvement is noted with cylinder correction, a spherical equivalent will suffice.

Low vision reading glasses may be prescribed as regular bifocals. This only is possible, however, in the lower powers. It is technically very difficult to place bifocal powers of higher than 6 D in the carrier lens of the distance correction. Check with the most experienced optician in your area to find out the limits of the local lab. Usually it is about 4 D to 6 D. Patients who can still read with standard style bifocals are very happy because their reading habits are relatively unchanged. The only change needed is a decrease in the reading distance relative to the new focal distance of the stronger reading add.

Beyond powers of 4 D to 6 D, single vision reading glasses become necessary. Because the reading distance is so much closer, patients have to converge excessively and no longer look through the optical centers of the lenses. Therefore, a base-in prism is included to offset the opti-

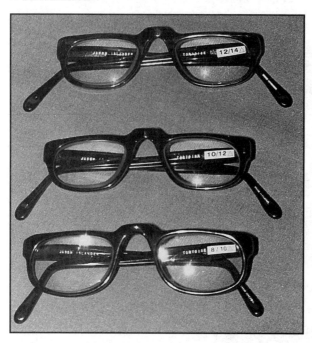

Figure 2-4. Half-eye spectacles with base-in prism already incorporated to facilitate binocular use.

cal centers and relieve the convergence demand. Stock binocular low vision reading glasses already have prism included (Figure 2-4). Six-diopter spectacles incorporate 8 prism D of base-in prism, 8-D lenses have 10 prism D base-in, and 10-D glasses have 12 D of base-in prism. These reading glasses are in the half-eye style so the patient can look above them for distance viewing.

Above powers of 12 D, spectacles are referred to as microscopes, and are usually supplied in full-frame spectacles rather than half-eyes. They must be removed for distance viewing. It is better to recommend monocular low vision microscopes for just the preferred eye. The other eye is ignored while reading. This allows the patient to focus at very close distances without the need to converge. (Sometimes a patient may experience difficulty with binocularity even at the lower powers. Reading lenses of any power may be supplied for only one eye instead of binocularly. An alternative method of dealing with binocular problems is to suggest that a monocular occluder be worn over the least preferred eye.)

There are advantages to using spectacles as low vision aids. Primarily, patients are used to them. They are comfortable, common, have no stigma attached, and adaptation is easy. They allow both hands to be free for holding books, menus, newspapers, etc. Because they are worn on the face or can be strung on a neck chain, they are not as easily misplaced as handheld devices. Insurance sometimes covers spectacles if the patient has a vision-care rider, while magnifiers rarely are covered by third-party payers.

The disadvantages of spectacles occur when higher powers are needed. The reading distance becomes abnormally close and patients find it difficult to adjust. Depth of field also becomes narrower with high powers, rendering it difficult to maintain the point of focus. Also, holding reading material close to the face blocks available light, thereby diminishing contrast and reducing the ability to see.

When these problems become pronounced, it may be time to try alternative magnifiers. One option is to try telemicroscopes, sophisticated magnifying systems only prescribed by experienced low vision providers. They are spectacles that have a telescope built right into the lens. When focused for near they provide high magnification powers but allow a longer, more func-

What the Patient Needs to Know

- When using spectacles, reading material must be held at the focusing distance of the lenses, which is *closer* to the eyes than normal. Touch the reading material to your nose and *slowly* move it away until it is in clear focus. Maintain that distance while reading.

- It may help to move reading material from side to side, keeping the eyes still, instead of scanning material in the normal way by moving your eyes from the beginning to the end of a line of print.

tional working distance. (A more complete discussion of telemicroscopes is found in the section on telescopes in this chapter.)

Patient Instruction With Spectacles

When spectacles are prescribed as low vision aids, it is necessary to inform the patient of the optical principles and all the disadvantages. Low vision assistants should instruct patients in several areas. The most important is reading distance. If someone is prescribed a 16 D spectacle add, his or her vision will be blurry at the previously preferred "normal" working distance. The best way to teach adaptation to short focal lengths is to have the patient touch his or her nose with the reading material, then slowly back it away until it comes into focus. Because each patient's initial reaction is to move reading material *away* to focus better, this technique is the most satisfactory. If the patient starts with the print too far away, it is very difficult for him or her to adapt to pulling it closer to focus. The patient will become frustrated and possibly give up trying.

The second issue is that some distortion occurs when moving the eyes from side to side. This is more pronounced in the higher power lenses. When this problem occurs, a constant and clearer image is possible if the head is kept still and the paper is moved from side to side. This is a difficult adjustment to make and will require patience of the instructor and the patient.

Assistants should also discuss lighting needs with patients. This issue is discussed more fully in the section in this chapter on nonoptical low vision aids.

Hand Magnifiers

Hand magnifiers consist of a convex lens surrounded by a plastic or metal carrier attached to a handle (Figure 2-5). Sometimes they have a light attached. Hand magnifiers are commonly prescribed for low vision patients. They are readily available in most hardware and drug stores, and many patients pick them up independently to try to improve reading. The optical principles of hand magnifiers are based on the same rules as spectacles, but introduce another concept. Because the lens is not worn on the face, there is now an eye-to-magnifier distance as well as a magnifier-to-print distance.

For maximum magnification with a hand magnifier, hold the lens a distance from the reading material that is equal to the focal distance of the lens. For example, hold an 8-D magnifier 12.5 cm from the print (100 cm ÷ 8 D = 12.5 cm focal distance). Hold a 20-D magnifier 5 cm from the print (100 cm ÷ 20 D = 5 cm focal distance). This is the same calculation used to determine the reading distance for a patient wearing high power spectacles. Changing the magnifier-to-print distance still will provide magnification, but it will not be optimal. The image size will be smaller and resolution will diminish.

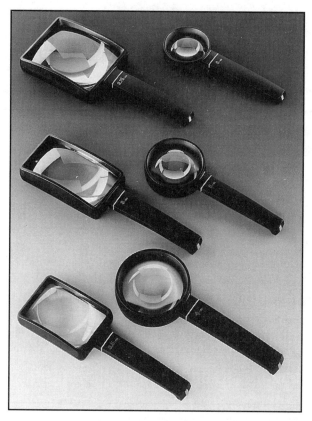

Figure 2-5. Hand magnifiers (photo courtesy Eschenbach Optik of America, Ridgefield, Conn).

When holding the magnifier at the proper lens-to-print distance (which is equal to the focal length of the lens) the image viewed by the eye will maintain a constant size. Moving the eye very close to the magnifier or very far away changes neither the size nor the focus. This is because rays of light from the magnifier emerge parallel to each other (Figure 2-6). They are not converging or diverging in relation to one another, so there is no focal point on the "back" side of the lens (the side facing toward the eyes). No accommodation is needed to focus the image and no reading correction is necessary. Patients who use hand magnifiers should view the image through the *distance* portion of their bifocals or when otherwise corrected to emmetropia at distance. Using a reading correction does not improve the focus or the magnification of the image. It will make both worse.

Changing the eye-to-magnifier distance does not affect focus or accommodative demand, but it can change the field of view. By moving the eye closer to the lens, the field will increase in size. This technique allows more words to be seen without moving the lens. Patients who constantly bring the magnifier to the eye for a larger field of view must be reminded about keeping the lens-to-print distance constant. In other words, they must bring the reading material closer to the eye at the same rate in which they bring the magnifier closer. They may eventually prefer a spectacle correction or loupe instead, as these lenses are already designed to be held at the plane of the eye.

Hand magnifiers are excellent for situations when the near material is at a fixed distance and cannot be brought closer to the eye. For instance, in a grocery store a magnifier can be used to look at labels of cans on the top shelf. Looking at temperature dials on a hot stove (Figure 2-7) or viewing a seam while machine sewing are other excellent uses. Hand magnifiers are extremely portable, so they are useful in any situation that requires a quick look. Reading price tags while shopping, looking up phone numbers in the telephone directory, and looking at photographs of

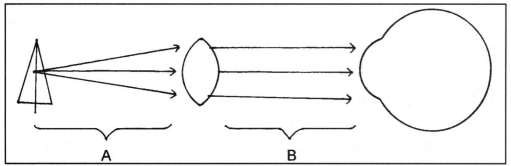

Figure 2-6. If the lens-to-object distance (A) is equal to the focal length of the lens, the emergent rays are parallel. Then the eye-to-lens distance (B) is variable.

What the Patient Needs to Know

- The distance from a hand magnifier to the printed page must be kept constant. To find this distance, start with the lens on the page and *slowly* pull it away from the print until optimal focus is reached.

- Hand magnifiers should be used with *distance* glasses.

- If the magnifier is brought closer to your eye to increase the field of view, bring the reading material closer as well. The distance from print to lens must always be kept constant to maintain focus.

the grandchildren are all good examples. The magnifier can be produced from a pocket or purse and returned just as quickly. A magnifier also can be used for long-term reading, but most patients find it difficult to handhold them at the correct focal distance for long periods. Because one hand-holds the aid, it is difficult to hold a book *and* turn pages with the other hand. A reading stand often is necessary.

The necessity to maintain a constant magnifier-to-print distance is the biggest disadvantage of hand magnifiers. Patients who lack arm strength or those with hand tremors find them difficult to use. Many patients inadvertently move the aid further from or closer to the page, with a subsequent loss of image clarity and magnification. Also, the hand that holds the lens and the lens carrier itself create shadows on the printed page and block out available light. This problem is exacerbated as the power increases and the magnifier-to-print distance is reduced.

Hand magnifiers come in many style variations for specific uses. These are mostly designed to eliminate some of the aforementioned disadvantages. One type hangs on a neckstrap and has a chest support to allow both hands freedom of movement for sewing or crafts. Another type is a large rectangular lens supported on a reading light so a book can be held beneath it and the light kept constant. Some are in small leather cases that flip open and can easily be carried in a pocket. There is probably a hand magnifier for most any use, and of any power your patient desires.

Patient Instruction With Hand Magnifiers

When patients begin to use hand magnifiers, the tendency is to hold the lens up to the eye and look through it. They do not seem to grasp the idea of holding the magnifier near the page and maintaining the longer reading distance. To make it clear, have your patients start with the mag-

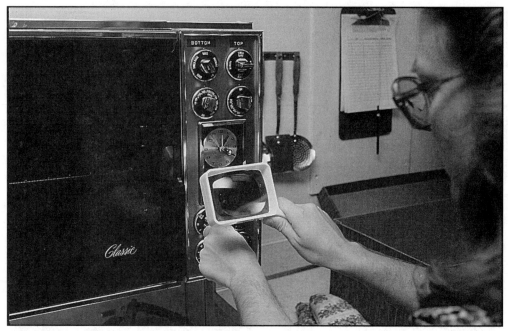

Figure 2-7. A hand magnifier has many helpful uses in the home.

nifier flat on the page. They should then raise it slowly until the magnification is maximum. Have them repeat this process several times until they are familiar with the correct focal distance. Frequently repeat the idea of keeping this distance constant. Only after it is clear should you begin a discussion of field of view and changing the eye-to-magnifier distance. Patients easily confuse the two concepts.

Reinforce the fact that distance glasses should be worn while using hand magnifiers. Elderly patients are used to thinking in terms of using bifocals for near work. They have a hard time adjusting to this change.

When discussing lighting, recommend a style of lamp that can be positioned to direct light onto the paper *underneath* the lens. Magnifiers with built-in light sources are accepted quickly and preferred by many people.

Unlike spectacles, hand magnifiers can easily be moved across a line of print without distortion. It is not necessary to move the book beneath the lens. In some inexpensive models there is distortion around the periphery of the lens. Aspheric magnifiers eliminate this problem by changing the power as the glass recedes away from the optical center. This manufacturing "trick" provides a clear focus across the entire lens. Most magnifiers offered by low vision suppliers are aspheric, so distortion is minimal.

Stand Magnifiers

Stand magnifiers are similar to hand magnifiers. They consist of a convex lens surrounded by a plastic or metal carrier (Figure 2-8). Instead of a handle, however, they are attached to legs or some other support. These enable the magnifier to stand freely on a page of print. Some have an internal light source, and some are moderately focusable by screwing the lens closer to or further from the page. Focusing does not affect magnification significantly, but can correct for moderate refractive errors of the user's eye.

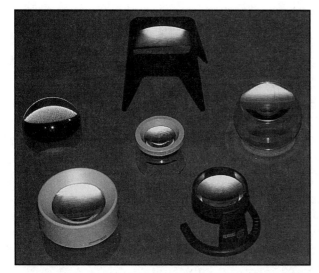

Figure 2-8. Stand magnifiers.

The legs of most stand magnifiers are shorter than the focal length of the lens to provide portability and a clear image to the periphery of the lens. As a result, image rays emerging from the back of the lens are not parallel. They are still somewhat divergent, making the image appear to come from a point further away than the actual location (a virtual image). Before viewing by the eye, these divergent rays must be focused. This can be accomplished by using accommodation or by viewing through reading glasses or the reading segment of a bifocal. The bifocal power should be determined for the focal distance of the virtual image (Figure 2-9). Because this virtual image is further away than the actual image, the effective magnification is less. Stand magnifiers do not achieve maximum magnification from the power of their lenses. This means that the power listed in catalogues is not equivalent to the actual magnification achieved. For this reason, a higher power of stand magnifier will be necessary to achieve the same level of reading comfort as a lower power hand magnifier or spectacles.

With stand magnifiers, the magnifier-to-print distance is constantly maintained by the legs of the apparatus. It is not necessary for the patient to worry about controlling focal length, so many patients prefer stand rather than hand magnifiers. Elderly patients adapt more easily because bifocals or reading glasses are worn. It is a familiar situation for near vision and few habits need to be changed.

The eye-to-lens distance must be fairly constant and depends on the power of the bifocal. Stronger reading adds allow closer working distances and provide somewhat higher magnification. These distances are much less variable than a hand magnifier and the field of view can be only minimally improved by moving nearer to the lens. The image will simply go out of focus unless a stronger reading add is employed.

One disadvantage of stand magnifiers is lack of portability. Many are small enough to be carried in a purse but not a pocket, as most styles do not fold or collapse. They can be cumbersome and rarely have cases, so the lens can scratch easily. The patient is better served using one on a desk or table. A supplementary hand magnifier for use outside the home is usually necessary.

Stand magnifiers also limit the amount of light that falls on the reading material. Because the lens and carrier is very close to the page, a shadow is cast directly on the print. The support stand itself also blocks light from entering at the sides. Light that comes directly through the lens is focused, creating a spot of light smaller than the field of view. The resultant brightness and shadow creates an intriguing test of patience and ingenuity to read or maneuver a light

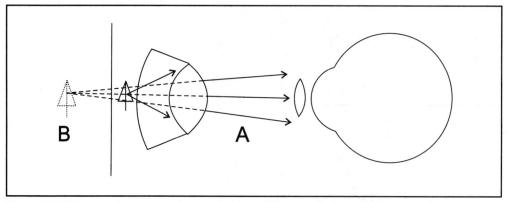

Figure 2-9. Light rays that emerge from a stand magnifier are divergent (A), so a reading correction is necessary to focus the virtual image (B).

What the Patient Needs to Know

- Wear your bifocals, reading glasses, or other near correction when using a stand magnifier. You will feel a "pull" on your eyes if you try to use the portion of your glasses that is for driving and watching television.
- Always keep the distance from your eyes to the magnifier constant. Do not pull the magnifier up to your eye or the focus will be lost.

source through the legs and onto the print. Designers have tried many tricks to solve this problem. Some stand magnifiers are attached to flashlights or other light sources (Figure 2-10). Others have wider spaces between narrower legs or have clear plastic housings that allow light to pass through all sides.

Reading a book can be difficult because the binding at the junction of two pages sometimes prevents the stand from moving all the way to the end of the print on the left page, or the beginning of the print on the right page. Stand magnifiers also have a relatively limited field of view. For all these reasons, stand magnifiers are best used for tasks such as hobbies. *Spotting*, which is looking at a subject in one location, is more suited to stand magnifiers than long-term reading, where the magnifier must be moved across lines and columns of print. Movement of a magnifier during use is referred to as *scanning*.

Patient Instruction With Stand Magnifiers

Patients with tremors or lack of arm control enjoy stand magnifiers because the lens-to-print distance is constantly provided by the stand itself. Older patients require very little instruction in spectacle correction because reading glasses are used. This is normal and acceptable to most patients.

The eye-to-lens distance causes some difficulty and requires explanation. Patients like to pull stand magnifiers up to their eyes as if viewing through a telescope. This will improve the field of view only minimally, and blur the image if accommodation is inadequate. Instruct your patients to maintain an appropriate reading distance. The ideal length is slightly shorter than the focal length of the bifocal. If your patient is a young person with high accommodative reserves, closer distances are acceptable. If a patient persists in holding a stand magnifier close to the eye, suggest high power spectacles instead. They achieve the same purpose, and keep the hands free.

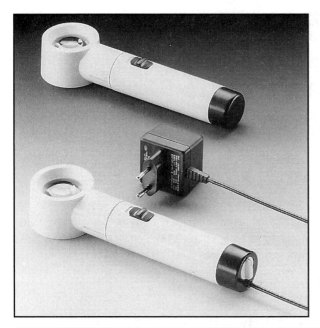

Figure 2-10. Lighted stand magnifiers (photo courtesy of Eschenbach Optik of America).

What the Patient Needs to Know

- Clean the lenses of low vision aids with a soft cloth and lens cleaning solution or water.

- Store lenses in their cases or wrapped in a soft cloth, as they tend to scratch very easily.

The more creative you are, the more you will be able to help your patients with the lighting dilemma. A gooseneck or moveable arm lamp is mandatory to shine light on the print yet underneath the lens. Some low vision providers remove one or more of the legs, allowing a larger window for the light to enter. Removing legs in this way also helps with the problem of the bookbinding impeding movement of the lens to the end of the print. It is tricky to provide larger light openings while maintaining stability of the base. The design of Combined Optical Industries Ltd. (COIL) brand magnifiers (Slough, Berkshire, United Kingdom) has been altered to reduce this problem by removing one edge of the base. Other manufacturers will probably follow suit.

Loupes

Loupes are high plus (convex) lenses that are handheld close to the eye, worn on the head, or attach directly to existing spectacles (Figure 2-11). Sometimes they have a carrier that slides over or clips on the glasses, such as a jeweller's loupe. Other loupes are on a hinged arm that attaches to the temple of the spectacle frames. The loupe is lowered in front of the eye when additional power is needed. When it is no longer needed it is flipped out of the visual axis.

Loupes are used in the same way as high power spectacles. They require a short eye-to-print distance that shortens as the power increases. The convenient aspect of a loupe is the ability to attach or detach it at will. They are convenient, lightweight, and available in many strengths. They are best when used for very close viewing, as in examining photographs, coins, or other small objects.

The disadvantages of loupes are the short working distance and a reduced field of view through the small diameter lenses. Spectacle attachments usually are less than ideal as well. The

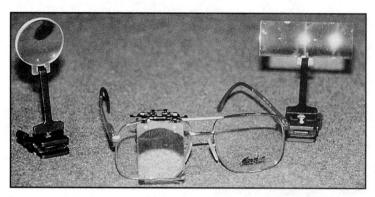

Figure 2-11. Spectacle-mounted loupes.

clip-on types tend to slip off center, and the moveable-arm types break easily. Also, as they only attach to one lens, the glasses may sit at a cockeyed angle and require more frequent adjustments. Varieties worn on the head are much more stable, but more bulky. Be sure to add the power of the spectacles to that of the loupe when determining focal distance.

Patient Instruction With Loupes

Patients should be taught how to clean the lenses (with water or lens cleaner only), how to store them (in a soft cloth or box), and how to attach them to spectacles. The eye-to-print distance must be kept constant in the same way as with spectacles.

Telescopes

Handheld

Telescopes (Figure 2-12) are more complex optical systems that consist of two lenses separated by a short distance in a metal tube. Astronomical telescopes are a common type, but cause the image to be viewed upside down. Galilean telescopes allow the image to be viewed upright, so they are the type most often used for low vision. In Galilean telescopes, a concave lens nearest the eye is called the *ocular* and a convex lens closer to the object being viewed is the *objective.* Sometimes a prism and mirror are incorporated in the carrier to decrease the distance between the lenses and render the telescope easier to hold in one hand. Low vision telescopes are minimally focusable. Some can be focused for distances as short as 2 ft to 3 ft, but most are for viewing objects across the room or at optical infinity. Telescopes are the only low vision aid that can be used to improve distance viewing.

Telescopes are labelled according to power and field of view. An 8 × 20, 7.5 monocular telescope indicates the following: The image seen through the telescope is 8 times larger than normal, or 8×. The objective lens is 20 mm in diameter, and the field of view is 7.5° through a normal size pupil.

Telescopes provide a clearer view by means of "angular magnification." This complex optical system results in divergent rays coming through the ocular lens that provide a larger retinal image. When using a telescope, the brain knows the actual distance of the object, so one cannot interpret the object as being larger. By experience, we know that objects decrease in size with distance, so large objects are interpreted as being closer. With either interpretation the result is the same—increased resolution of a distant object.

Telescopes have several shortcomings. As an image is viewed, there is a decrease in the amount of transmitted light, so the image will appear darker. Also, as the power increases, field of view

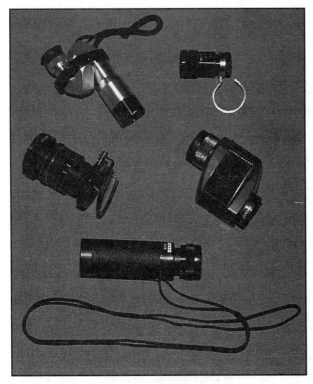

Figure 2-12. Handheld, spectacle-mounted, and finger-ring telescopes.

decreases dramatically. A larger field of view is possible with the use of binoculars instead of a monocular telescope. Some low power binoculars such as the COIL Spectacle Binocular® and Selsi (Midland Park, NJ) Sport Spectacles® are designed to be worn as glasses so they are relatively manageable. Other handheld types can be bulky so they are not as widely accepted as low vision aids. They are only used in special situations such as in a theater or at sporting events.

If a telescope is moved even slightly, the movement of the viewed image is magnified. A 5° movement of the user's hand is small, but the image will make a fast sweeping movement completely out of the small field of view. This is referred to as *motion parallax* and creates difficulty .in using handheld telescopes. It completely eliminates the use of a telescope while walking, driving, or otherwise moving. Arm fatigue and tremors also cause problems using handheld telescopes, so the weight of each type should be considered.

Bioptics

Bioptics are an alternative to the handheld variety of telescopes. These attach directly to spectacle lenses *above* the optical axis. The chin can be dipped down slightly, allowing the user to spot an object through the telescope, then walk toward it with head erect looking through the spectacle carrier lens as usual. Bioptics are excellent for mobility purposes. The telescope is used to sight bus numbers or street signs, but the glasses are used for safe walking with a wide field of view.

It is legal in 30 states and in Washington DC to drive using bioptic telescopes. The criteria for licensing varies in each state, but there are some general standards. In all but six of the states, the user must achieve 20/40 acuity through the bioptic. In no states are patients allowed to drive with bioptics if their regular best corrected visual acuity falls below the 20/200 level, and in most states it must be better than that. Visual field size also is a criteria for legal licensing with bioptics in most states.

Driving with bioptics has been controversial for many years. Some people cite the safety of society in trying to discourage people from driving with poor vision. The proponents, however,

---

What the Patient Needs to Know

- Telescopes must be balanced and held steady by resting your hand against your face, and your arm against your body or other support.

- To locate an object, first view it with your naked eye before lifting the telescope and spotting through it.

- Do not walk or move when viewing through a telescope.

- Objects seen through a telescope appear to be closer than they are.

---

cite the excellent functional ability of patients while using bioptics. The decision is a very individual one for the driver and for each state legislature. Check with your local bureau of licensing for regulations in your state.

Telemicroscopes

Telemicroscopes are telescopes mounted just *under* the optical center of the spectacle lens like a protruding bifocal. These systems are used for reading instead of for distance viewing (Figure 2-13). A small cap with a low power lens is attached to the objective to allow clear focus at a normal reading distance. The telescope provides the magnification, and the power of the reading cap determines the reading distance. For example, a +2.00 cap focuses at 50 cm. The depth of focus is decreased in telemicroscopes so the viewing distance must be critically maintained.

Telemicroscopes are ideal for school or desk work. The telescope alone can be used to see a chalkboard, clock, or overhead projector by tipping the chin up. Snapping the reading cap in place changes the focus to desk length for ease in taking notes or long-term reading. Students in the higher grades and college find telemicroscopes very helpful. Telemicroscopes have a number of successful vocational uses for occupations requiring long term near work with an extended working distance, such as computer use. Patients who use them may have different power reading caps for uses requiring several working distances.

High minus contact lenses worn under a high plus reading glass can provide patients with a makeshift full-field telescope. This is an option for the very motivated patient who is able to adjust to constant use of a telescope by one eye, ignoring its use when reading or walking.

Handheld telescopes should be provided to nearly every low vision patient. Even the patient with few low vision needs should receive some help with distance viewing. The simpler brands and lower powers are relatively inexpensive, so handheld telescopes are excellent for young children who may require frequent replacement of them from loss or damage. This encourages distant vision and the use of telescopes before the stigma of using them has a chance to affect interest. Most children love telescopes for television watching and "spying" out the window. They are ideal for use in school (Figure 2-14).

Two uses of telescopes are not intuitively evident. They can be used successfully by patients with nystagmus and those with narrow visual fields. Very few patients with nystagmus experience oscillopsia, or the apparent motion of objects. Most can see well as the eyes pass by the telescope's ocular. Many patients with nystagmus have a null point where the eye movements are minimal. Holding the eyes in the null position is second nature to most people with nystagmus, and telescope use is extremely successful in this position.

Patients with a very narrow visual field can turn the telescope around and view through the objective. The image then is minified, allowing more information to be viewed within the lim-

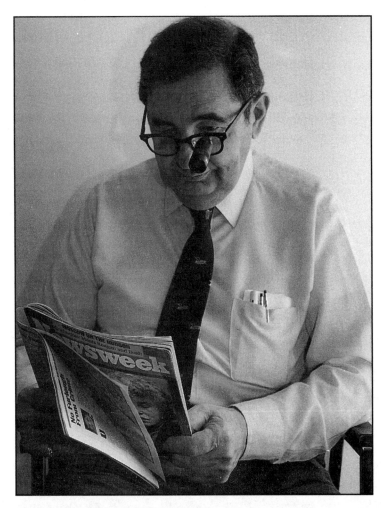

Figure 2-13. Telemicroscope for near use.

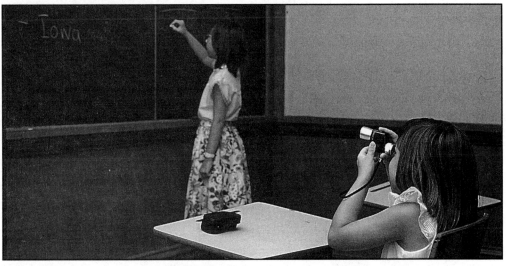

Figure 2-14. A young girl uses a handheld telescope in the classroom.

its of the patient's small visual field. For this technique, it is necessary that the patient's acuity is good enough to resolve the minified image. This often is the case in glaucoma and retinitis pigmentosa.

Patient Instruction With Telescopes

Telescopes are the most complex of all low vision aids and the most difficult to use correctly. Handheld varieties can and should be prescribed and taught by most low vision providers. Prescribing bioptics and telemicroscopes should only be attempted by experienced providers with a support staff of trained assistants including mobility instructors or occupational therapists. Such professionals are necessary to provide the follow-up training necessary for the successful use of these sophisticated devices.

Patients should be taught to use a telescope in several steps. First, the instructor should focus the telescope for infinity and teach the user the correct way to hold it (ie, with the ocular near the eye and the hand balanced against the face). Using two hands to hold the telescope provides more stability than one, and one arm or hand should be supported against a stationary object or the body. The patient should first view the distant object with the naked eye, then raise the telescope to view it more clearly. Always start with a well-lit object because the telescope blocks a great deal of light, and low contrast objects are thus very hard to see. Motion parallax will become evident very quickly, as well as the fact that objects appear to be much closer than they truly are. For these two reasons, instruct your patients not to attempt to walk while looking through the telescope. It should only be used while stationary.

After becoming proficient in spotting distant objects, your patient can be taught to change the focus for closer objects. Do this by picking out objects that are in the same line of view, both at least 15 ft away, and separated by at least 10 ft. Ask the patient to focus on the distant object, then view the nearer object, correcting the focus once it is in view. This should be practiced several times with different objects and varying distances. As practice progresses, the two chosen objects should be further apart. The most difficulty will be experienced when focusing from a very distant object to a very near one, or vice versa.

Once focusing is mastered, the patient can attempt scanning an area instead of only viewing a single object. This technique will be used when trying to take in a large field of view such as when watching sporting events or when trying to locate a person in a large room or field. The patient will learn to scan very slowly in order to overcome motion parallax and blurring. Instruct the patient to practice moving the telescope and his or her head as one unit. To practice the skill, several pictures or objects may be placed around a room, and the patient can be instructed to move his or her attention from one to the other. At first, the object should be placed at equal distances from the patient. As proficiency is gained some of the target objects should be closer than others, so the patient has to scan and focus at the same time.

The final skill to learn is tracking, or following a moving target. This skill will be necessary for watching an airplane take off or land, a person running a race, or any other moving object. The head and telescope are moved as one unit at the same speed as the moving target. Begin practice by following slow targets such as the instructor walking slowly. Gradually increase the speed of the moving object as the patient becomes more proficient.

Spotting, focusing, scanning, and tracking should each be taught separately and time allowed to practice between each of the three tasks to develop proficiency. It may require several visits before the individual becomes proficient with each of the skills, and can use the telescope efficiently.

Addresses of Low Vision Aid Vendors

Rather than providing the address of every vendor of low vision aids, the following two addresses should provide you with a wide variety of styles. Both of these vendors sell aids from most suppliers:

Lighthouse Low Vision Products
36-20 Northern Boulevard
Long Island City, NY 11101-1614
1-800-453-4923
Fax: 1-718-786-0437

Mattingly International, Incorporated
938-K Andreasen Drive
Escondido, CA 92029
1-800-826-4200

Bibliography

Faye E, Hood C. *Low Vision*. Springfield, Ill: Charles C. Thomas; 1975.

Fonda G. *Management of Low Vision*. New York, NY: Thieme-Stratton, Inc; 1981.

Jose R. *Understanding Low Vision*. New York, NY: American Foundation for the Blind; 1983.

Sloan L. *Recommended Aids for the Partially Sighted*. New York, NY: National Society for the Prevention of Blindness, Inc; 1971.

Wiener W, Vopata A. Suggested curriculum for distance training with optical aids. *The Journal of Visual Impairment and Blindness*. 1980;2:49-56.

Nonoptical and Electronic Low Vision Aids

- Nonoptical aids are available for reading, writing, medical use, and household use as well as for hobbies and games.

- Lighting is the most important nonoptical aid.

- Before using electronic aids, personal assessment and training should be undertaken in order to allow efficiency with the appliance.

Nonoptical Aids

A nonoptical low vision aid is any device other than a magnifier that enables partially sighted or blind individuals to function more easily in their daily tasks. This division of low vision aids includes items from a simple sewing needle threader that costs $1.00, to expensive electronic appliances. Each nonoptical aid has a specific use that enhances reading or tasks of daily living. A number of accessory devices provide increased contrast of reading materials. Other items incorporate larger print or are enlarged themselves, providing relative size magnification. Still others, such as audio or Braille versions of printed materials, provide assistance by avoiding visual limitations completely. Closed circuit televisions (CCTVs) magnify images with the use of video enlargement employing optical principles. As they are not optical aids in the usual sense, they are included in this Chapter with other electronic devices.

Many nonoptical devices have nothing to do with printed material. They assist with daily activities such as eating, food preparation, and household organization. Frequently they are just adaptations of ordinary objects to make them safer or more manageable for people hindered by subnormal vision.

There are too many nonoptical aids to mention individually, but an overview of the most common types follows.

Lighting

Light is the primary and most crucial nonoptical device. Contrast sensitivity fails as acuity decreases, and low vision patients must find a way to improve contrast of written materials to see them more easily. Most patients quickly realize that vision improves in sunlight, and independently install higher watt lightbulbs in their lamps. This increased illumination is functional but not ideal. In order to be most effective, light must be strong enough to provide maximum contrast without bleaching out the print or causing glare. For most patients, a 60-watt bulb is ideal for optimum contrast. Lower powers do not provide enough light, and higher powers cause glare. The bulb is best placed in a cone-shaped, reflective shade that directs 100% of the available light onto the page.

The arm of an ideal reading lamp must be a gooseneck or moveable type that allows the light to be shone directly onto the page of print (Figure 3-1). The arm of the lamp must have several moveable joints allowing the shade to be brought very close to the reading material and angled precisely to eliminate shadows.

These lamps are available widely in office supply stores. The least expensive varieties are fine for most uses, but higher priced varieties have the advantage of an insulated shade. This insulated shade is better for patients who view objects very close to their face and stay in close proximity to the lamp for a long time. The insulation keeps the shade cooler and helps prevent burns. Elderly patients need to be reassured that this close light source will not harm their eyes. They must also be re-educated that the old adage, "light must come over the left shoulder when reading," is a myth.

A good catalogue distributor of reading lamps for low vision is:
Lighting Specialties Company
735 Hastings Lane
Buffalo Grove, IL 60089
1-800-729-3366

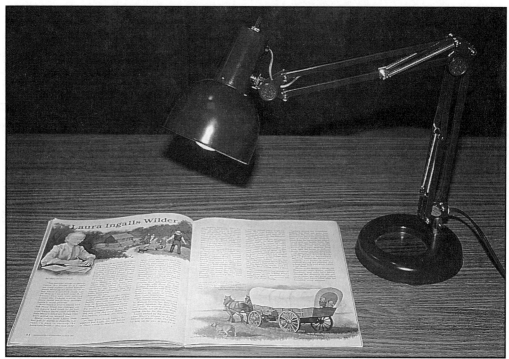

Figure 3-1. A reading lamp should have a flexible arm to enable the light to be directed from any user preferred angle.

Not all patients benefit from a direct light source. It is important to experiment with illumination positions and styles for each individual to determine what is optimal for each patient. Patients with ocular albinism or aniridia, or diabetics who have undergone laser therapy have light-sensitive retinas. Moveable arm lamps are still the best choice, but will be more useful if moved further from the page to decrease the light level. These patients also benefit from other nonoptical aids such as sunglasses and absorptive filters.

Special sunglasses that wrap around the patient's face and filter light from all angles are popular with low vision patients (Figure 3-2). Solarshields® (Dioptics Medical Products, San Luis Obispo, Calif) and NoIR (NoIR Medical Technologies, South Lyon, Mich) sunglasses are the best known varieties. Their design prevents glare in most light situations. Levels of protection vary from light tints with only ultraviolet protection to the most dense tints that allow transmission of only 2% of available light. Green or brown tints are good for decreasing light levels and to eliminate glare. Yellow enhances contrast and is useful for improving the readability of printed material, particularly blue ink. School children may use them to improve contrast of mimeographed sheets at school. A piece of letter-size yellow acetate film placed on mimeographed paper provides the same service if a child does not want to wear unusual sunglasses. Optical shops can tint the patient's standard prescription lenses for increased contrast or light protection as well.

Absorptive filter lenses are recommended particularly for patients with albinism, retinitis pigmentosa, macular degeneration, and glaucoma. Patients who have undergone cataract extraction or retinal laser treatment also benefit from their use. Some patients prefer light tints for indoors and darker tints for outdoors. Visors or hats with wide brims also protect the eyes from the brightness of the sun, and can increase visual efficiency outdoors.

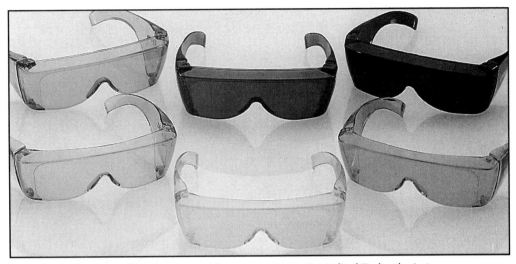

Figure 3-2. Absorptive filter sunglasses (photo courtesy NoIR Medical Technologies).

Order catalogues for absorptive sunglasses from:

NoIR Medical Technologies
PO Box 159
South Lyon, MI 48178
1-800-521-9746

Dioptics Medical Products
51 Zaca Lane #150
San Luis Obispo, CA 93401
1-800-959-9040
Fax: 1-805-781-3322

Patients with peripheral retinal degenerations may become debilitated in low light situations and become essentially "night blind." Night vision spotting scopes, designed for the Army, detect infrared light and make a scene appear bright even in very low light conditions. These are available as small handheld scopes or scopes worn on the head to help patients see at night or when entering a darkened room.

Reading and Writing Aids

"Large print" is a term that applies to any size print larger than the standard. In books, magazines, and newspapers large print generally refers to 18- or 24-point type, which is 2× magnification, or twice the size of "regular" print. The United States Postal Service uses 18-point type as their official size for large print that can be mailed without postage as "free matter for the blind."

Large-print books, magazines, and newspapers are widely available. They can eliminate the need for optical devices for patients with moderately low vision, and may be the only reading material possible for those with severe vision loss who use strong magnifiers. Local libraries carry many bestsellers and popular titles in large print. Several agencies such as the National Library Service for the Blind and Physically Handicapped, and the National Association for the Visually Handi-

---

What the Patient Needs to Know

- Brighter lightbulbs are not the only answer to help you read better. Sometimes a lower watt bulb is better. In either case, the illumination should shine directly on the subject matter.

- Light can be placed in any location that provides optimal contrast of the print. It is not necessarily best if it comes over your shoulder from behind.

- Bright light on a page of print will not harm your eyes.

- If glare is a problem for you, it is okay to move your reading light further away or wear sunglasses indoors.

Visually Handicapped (NAVH) (address on page 42) have large print lending libraries that can be accessed through the mail. Most reference books such as dictionaries and atlases are commercially available in large-print editions as well. *The New York Times*® is published weekly in a condensed version in large print, and magazines such as the *Reader's Digest*® and *Newsweek*® are also available (Figure 3-3).

National Library Service for the Blind and Physically Handicapped
The Library of Congress
1291 Taylor Street NW
Washington DC 20542
1-202-707-5100

The New York Times Large Type Weekly
PO Box 9564
Uniondale, NY 11555
1-800-631-2580

Reader's Digest Large Type Association
PO Box 241
Mt. Morris, IL 61054
1-800-877-5293

Most school textbooks are available in, or can be converted to, large print or Braille. Contact:

American Printing House for the Blind
PO Box 6085
Louisville, KY 40206
1-800-223-1839
Fax: 1-502-899-2274

Regular personal computer software allows choices of font size so manuscripts and term papers can easily be converted from small to large print and back again. Teachers can provide assignments and classroom materials in large print for their visually impaired students when the

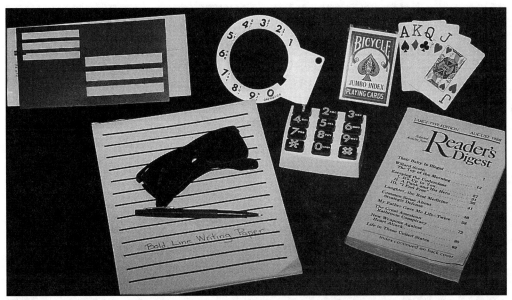

Figure 3-3. Large print and other nonoptical low vision aids. Clockwise from upper left, envelope addressing stencil, large print telephone dial, large print playing cards, large-print *Reader's Digest®*, large print touch-tone phone dial, bold line writing paper with black felt-tip pen, NoIR absorptive sunglasses.

papers are prepared on computers. There are also special computer programs that allow the entire screen to be seen in larger print sizes. These programs are discussed further in the section on electronic appliances at the end of this chapter. Computers can be used with moderately limited vision without any alterations or special programs simply by buying a larger monitor. A 21-inch monitor already enlarges the entire screen to the equivalent of large print while providing a full field of view. Special computer screen magnifiers that attach to regular size monitors are also available.

Line isolators (typoscopes) are cardboard strips with rectangular sections cut out which isolate one or two lines of print on a page. These eliminate all distracting background print when reading or writing. They are commercially available or may be homemade of laminated black construction paper or posterboard. Some are pocket size with an opening only big enough for a signature, and allow patients to "sign on the dotted line" without having to see the dotted line. Some are cut as stencils for addressing envelopes or writing checks.

Reading stands sit on a table or desk and hold reading material at a proper height and angle. They promote a more comfortable posture for the very close reading distances necessary when using low vision aids. They also support the book, freeing one hand for reading with a magnifier (Figure 3-4). A reading lamp can be situated next to a reading stand so the optimum light is always available where it is needed. Many patients find this system invaluable in reducing stress and effort when reading with optical low vision aids. There are many styles of reading stands commercially available, or patients can build their own if they prefer a simpler design.

Black felt-tip markers draw lines that are read more easily than those from pens and pencils. Low vision patients should keep a supply on hand and instruct their friends and family members to use them in correspondence. Low vision supply vendors also sell bold-lined writing paper which is lined like notebook paper, but with bold black lines. School children find this very helpful when learning to write, as the lines on standard writing tablets have very low contrast and are extremely difficult to see.

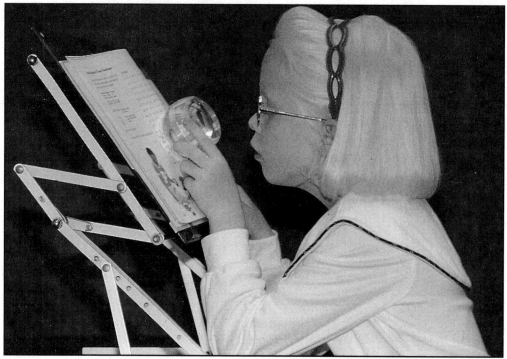

Figure 3-4. A reading stand holds material at the proper angle for use with magnifiers.

Medical Devices

Many medical devices have been adapted to enable low vision patients to remain involved in their own care, particularly diabetics. There are syringes with magnifiers attached or with large-print numbers on the syringe itself. Blood sugar monitors are available with attachable voice synthesizers that speak the readout. Adapters for medicine vials ensure that the needle passes through the center of the rubber stopper without bending or breaking. There are also talking blood pressure cuffs and thermometers, and other large print medical items.

Household Appliances

Nonoptical aids for the home include large-print or Braille clocks and watches, talking calculators, and large print telephone dials for rotary or push-button phones. Cooking appliances vary from a knife with a detachable guide for measuring slices of bread, to complete sets of dishes with rims to allow patients to push their food on their plates without pushing it off the edges. Talking egg timers and safety accessories for ironing are just a few of the hundreds of other household appliances available.

Hobbies and Games

For sewing enthusiasts there are appliances that help thread needles and tape measures with tactile dots to help with accurate measuring. For woodworkers, most tools have adaptations to aid in measuring, cutting, and protection. Game players can enjoy their favorite games such as Monopoly®, Bingo®, or Backgammon® with the aid of large print and Braille versions (Figure 3-5). Playing cards come in large-print styles, as do crossword puzzles and the game of Scrabble®.

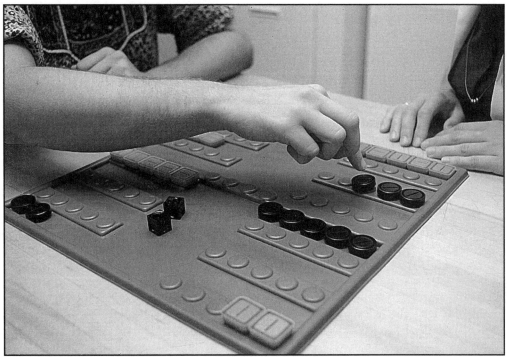

Figure 3-5. A tactile Backgammon® game can be enjoyed by sighted or blind players.

Sports enthusiasts can play their favorite sports with the aid of "beep balls." These are standard basketballs and soccer balls, as well as play footballs and various size foam balls, that are supplied with internal bells or electronic beepers to aid in localization while playing.

Braille

Usually low vision providers think in terms of providing larger print or higher power magnifiers to patients. It is easy to forget that there is a time when Braille becomes the best choice, or even an alternate one for written communication. The six dots that compose the Braille "alphabet" were devised by Louis Braille, a blind musician and gifted student in France in the mid-19th century. A similar code started as a method of night communication for Louis XVIII's Army, but was transformed as a code of writing for blind students by Louis Braille.[1] The dotted "code" spread quickly for use as a means of written communication by blind people across the world. The six dots in a Braille cell (two across, three down) are arranged in various combinations, each of which stands for a letter, number, or group of letters such as "ing" or "tion." Books and magazines are available in Braille for adults and children, and unavailable titles and texts can be converted to Braille. Conversion is time-consuming, so orders for specific school texts must be submitted far in advance of when classes begin. Teachers and parents need to plan ahead. Contact the American Printing House for the Blind (address on page 34), or:

The National Braille Press
88 Saint Stephen Street
Boston, MA 02115
1-617-266-6160
Fax: 1-617-437-0456

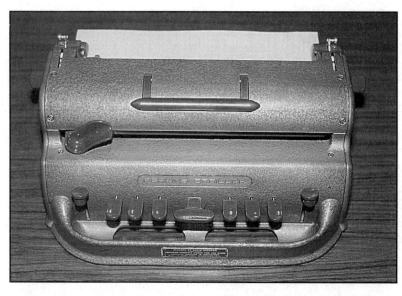

Figure 3-6. The Perkins Brailler embosses paper with Braille cells.

Braille is written with a rather cumbersome apparatus called a Braille Writer, (or Perkins Brailler), which looks and functions like a manual typewriter (Figure 3-6). For more portable writing, notes can be taken with the use of a small stencil and punch, called a "slate and stylus." With a Braille slate and stylus, metal Braille "stickers" can be individually punched and applied to games and appliances to orient blind individuals. For instance, the "on/off" and "volume" switches can be labelled on a stereo or compact disc player for easier location. Most of us have seen these stickers labelling the floor numbers near elevator buttons in public buildings.

Some patients find it difficult to differentiate the various Braille symbols. The dots are close together and are raised only slightly off the smooth paper. The fingers of some adult patients are too large to locate the small dots accurately. Diabetics have decreased sensation to their extremities and cannot sense the raised dots at all. Other patients simply cannot learn the new "language." Braille is not for everyone, but should not be forgotten as a possible and excellent alternative for some patients.

Electronic Devices and Computer-Assistive Technology

Like all electronic devices, those for use by visually impaired people continue to improve and become more compact each year. The best way to stay abreast of the technology is to contact manufacturing representatives regularly. Any specific device listed in this book may be outmoded at any time and should be investigated before suggesting it to patients. There are several categories of electronic assistive devices that are the most helpful.

Closed Circuit Televisions

CCTVs are used in visual rehabilitation. They consist of a video monitor with a small video camera attached beneath them or installed internally. Written material can be placed under the camera, where it is filmed instantly and transmitted onto the monitor in large print (Figure 3-7). The print size is variable and can be enlarged from 2× to so large it will allow only several characters on the screen at a time. As the print becomes larger the field of view becomes smaller, and

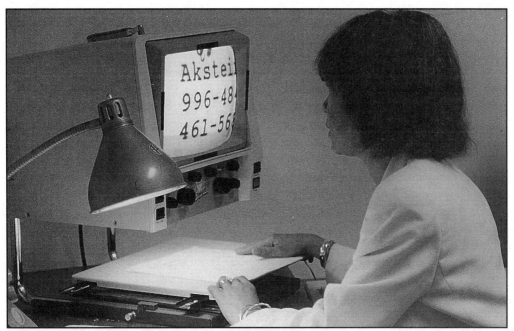

Figure 3-7. A closed circuit television in use at work.

sometimes tracking the page back and forth can cause smearing or jerking of the print. Slowing the tracking speed helps eliminate these difficulties. CCTVs enable patients to read materials that are not otherwise available in large print. They are excellent for viewing illustrations, photographs, or collectibles such as coins and stamps. They also come with attachments for typewriters and computer keyboards to assist in the workplace and at school. Some CCTVs can be electronically connected to computers to allow the image from a book to be viewed directly on the computer screen. The view from the CCTV can sometimes appear in a split screen, so that a word processing program can be viewed simultaneously for taking notes.

Computer Programs

Standard computers are useful for low vision patients when a large-size font is chosen. Some programs may be difficult to learn, however, because most of the setup literature and on-screen tollbars are too small to be seen. A better alternative is to use one of the specialized software packages designed for IBM compatible and MacIntosh computers. These software programs can be directly installed into a personal computer to allow the user to see most any other software program in larger print (Figure 3-8). The advantage to using this type of program over just using a larger font size is that the icons and toolbar are also seen in larger sizes. In addition, functions are included that are helpful in navigating around a document while only viewing a small portion of it. The print size can be changed from 2× to 16× at the touch of a key. These programs can be used with current word processing programs, accounting programs, the Internet, and E-mail.

Synthesized Speech

A voice synthesizer is another type of adaptive device that is useful, particularly for patients with severe visual loss. These devices convert the printed word to synthesized speech. Some systems directly attach to electronic appliances such as clocks and thermometers to "speak" the dig-

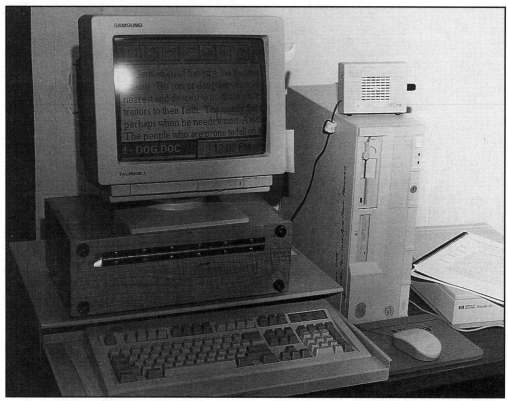

Figure 3-8. The installation of a large print software program allows this computer to present other programs and their tool bars in larger type.

ital readout. They can also attach to computers, and some are included in computer software packages. This is the only method of adapting laptop computers, as they do not have monitors big enough to accommodate a larger print size.

These synthesized speech devices can be set to speak each letter as it is typed or to read entire words. The voice is easy to understand and accurate in pronunciation. Speech-adapted computers are excellent for patients with severe disabilities. They also are good for patients with better vision but for whom computer-induced eye fatigue is a problem. Other voice synthesizers, such as the Xerox Imaging System® (Xerox Imaging Systems, Peabody, Mass) looks like a small photocopier. It can scan an entire page of printed material and read it aloud or transfer it to a computer screen.

For Braille users, there are computer adaptations that incorporate Braille into the system. Some keyboards have "refreshable" Braille components. This is a small section below the keypad that has a number of small 6 dot Braille cells with movable pins in each cell. As words are printed on the screen, they are transposed to Braille and the appropriate pins stick up on the pad so the user can feel the Braille letters. There are also special printers that emboss Braille on heavier bond paper instead of printing typical characters with ink.

Large print and synthesized speech computer programs are available from:
A I Squared, Incorporated
PO Box 669
Manchester Center, VT 05255-0669
1-802-362-3612

Berkeley Systems Incorporated
2095 Rose Street
Berkeley, CA 94709-1720
1-510-540-5535
Fax: 1-510-540-5630 (general number)
Fax: 1-510-849-9426 (free catalogue)

Optelec US Incorporated
6 Lyberty Way
Westford, MA 01886
1-508-392-0707
Fax: 1-508-692-6073

Along with computers, CCTVs are available from:

HumanWare, Incorporated
6245 King Road
Loomis, CA 95650
1-800-722-3393

Telesensory
455 N Bernardo Avenue
Mountain View, CA 94043
1-800-227-8418
Fax: 1-415-969-9064

Synthesized speech systems are available from:

Blazie Engineering
105 E Jarrettsville Road
Forest Hill, MD 21050-1611
1-410-893-9333
Fax: 1-410-836-5040

Xerox Imaging Systems
9 Centennial Drive
Peabody, MA 01960
1-800-421-7323
Fax: 1-508-977-2148

Speech Compression

Tape recorders with "speech compression" play recorded information at a higher than normal speed, but in normal frequency so the speech sounds normal instead of like chipmunks. They are useful for students and office workers who must process a great deal of printed and spoken material. Students use them to replay lectures at high speed, pausing or marking an area with tone indexing when important material is covered. Notes can then be transposed onto computer or into

Braille notes. Sometimes textbooks or other materials are unavailable in large-print or recorded versions. Partially sighted students hire readers to speak the material onto audio tape. The tape can then be reviewed at normal or high speed. Listening at high speed takes some getting used to, but motivated students learn to rely on it heavily. Most recorders designed for the visually impaired have speech compression as a standard feature. Other standard recorders such as the Sony Walkman® can be adapted with a microchip to allow for speech compression capabilities.

The standard speech compression machines are distributed by the National Library Service for the Blind and Physically Handicapped (see page 34 for address) when patients enroll in the Talking Book program. Other recorders can be purchased from the American Printing House for the Blind (see page 34 for address).

Because low vision electronic adaptive technology changes as quickly as any other technology, it is very important for patients to receive some guidance when purchasing a program or device. Ideally, each patient should undergo an "assistive technology assessment" by an experienced instructor before attempting to purchase a computer program for home or work use. These assessments can be scheduled through the state agency for the blind in each state. If there are no services available locally, the American Foundation for the Blind (AFB) has a technology center that provides reviews of the latest products and help with deciding which device may be appropriate for particular tasks (call 1-800-232-5463). The AFB can also refer a patient to an agency in his or her local area to receive some individualized counselling. Training will prove to be invaluable to the user's efficiency with each device. The companies that market the devices do not offer this type of training and follow-up.

Nonoptical aids listed in this chapter that do not have specific addresses included can be ordered by catalogue from distributors who carry a large variety of aids. Order your free catalogues from the following:

"Products to Help People with Impaired Vision"
The Lighthouse, Incorporated
36-20 Northern Boulevard
Long Island City, NY 11101-1614
1-800-829-0500
Fax: 1-718-786-5620

LS&S Group, Incorporated
PO Box 673
Northbrook, IL 60065
1-800-468-4789

"Visual Aids Catalog"
National Association for Visually Handicapped (NAVH)
22 W 21st Street, 6th Floor
New York, NY 10010
1-212-889-3141

Independent Living Aids, Incorporated
27 East Mall
Plainview, NY 11803
1-800-537-2118

Reference

1.Wallechinsky D, Wallace I. The People's Almanac. Garden City, NY: Doubleday and Co; 1975:520-521.

Bibliography

McGillivray R. Comprehensive computer access evaluation for persons with low vision. *Aids and Appliances Review*. 1994;15:2-8.

Stetten D. Sounding board: coping with blindness. *New Engl J Med*. 1981;305:458-460.

Chapter 4

History Taking

KEY POINTS

- A low vision history should address rehabilitation as well as optical concerns.

- A low vision exam and history should not be attempted until the patient has reached a level of acceptance of his or her visual loss.

- A well-informed patient experiences more success with low vision aids.

- Teacher input should be solicited for the history of school-age patients.

Role of Patient History in Low Vision

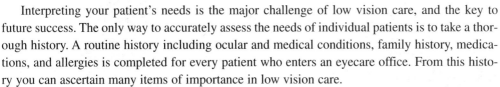

Interpreting your patient's needs is the major challenge of low vision care, and the key to future success. The only way to accurately assess the needs of individual patients is to take a thorough history. A routine history including ocular and medical conditions, family history, medications, and allergies is completed for every patient who enters an eyecare office. From this history you can ascertain many items of importance in low vision care.

The patient's ocular diagnosis provides immediate insight into the direction you may be taking. For instance, patients with macular degeneration will have central scotomas and require magnification for reading and other near tasks. They also have a progressive disease requiring more frequent follow-up care to assess their changing needs.

The medical history provides valuable information as well (Figure 4-1). For example, insulin-dependent diabetics experience frequent fluctuations in their acuity. Several powers of low vision aids may be necessary for these patients to use as their blood sugar levels rise and fall. If they have undergone laser surgery, diabetic retinopathy patients are light sensitive and you must address their specific lighting needs. Usually they prefer more diffuse light than other visually impaired patients, and will also benefit from counselling about different sunglasses and absorptive filters.

Although this routine ocular or medical history is imperative, it is not the whole story. A history for a low vision patient is more comprehensive. The four major goals are to:
1. Ascertain the visual expectations and needs of the patient
2. Determine the patient's acceptance of the visual loss and realistic understanding of the prognosis
3. Learn what social support system is in place through family, friends, or agencies
4. Create rapport and win the patient's trust

Ascertain the Visual Expectations and Needs of the Adult Patient

The visual expectations of the patient are not always realistic. For instance, a patient with severe visual loss and narrow visual field secondary to glaucoma may want to drive. When you ask what visual tasks have been given up and which are the most important to this patient, the first response will be "I want to drive again." Older people with vision loss usually want their vision restored to its former level. They want to drive, read, play cards, and be totally independent. Moreover, they want to achieve those goals by having their vision restored to its former level. They may enter the low vision exam with unrealistic expectations. It is the job of the history taker to narrow these expectations to an achievable level.

Goals can be narrowed without discouraging the patient. For instance, if the patient desires to drive, you can sympathize and say you understand that lack of freedom of mobility is difficult. At this time you don't know of any states that would allow this patient to receive a driver's license. There are alternatives however, and you are willing to work to restore some of his or her former independence. Ask your patient if there is a city bus line near his or her home or a senior center that offers transportation. If the patient is unaware of any local transportation, a referral to a social agency will be in order. The fear of travelling with public transportation might be related to an inability to see well enough to read bus stop signs. Sometimes the inability to read a

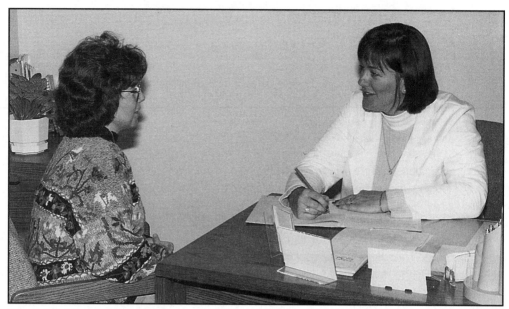

Figure 4-1. History taking allows you to develop a rapport with patients and determine their needs, desires, and concerns.

watch might inhibit a person from using buses for fear of missing the scheduled pickup and becoming stranded. A handheld telescope and a mobility lesson concerning bus routes might relieve the first fear, while a talking or large-print watch would relieve the second fear.

Conversely, low vision patients may have their expectations set too low. They may have tried a magnifier in the past without success and feel sure that you cannot help them in any way. They are frequently unaware of services and aids that are available. It is necessary for the person taking the history to ask leading questions about specific vocational needs or hobbies. Also inquire about requirements for distance viewing other than driving, and activities of daily living that have become difficult. You might question what usually is eaten for dinner, how it is cooked or prepared, what problems arise in using the stove, and how food shopping is done. Some patients eat cold cereal and packaged food because of an inability to see the dials on the stove or fear of starting a fire. Marking the stove dials with tactile dots to locate various temperature settings can remedy this problem. Grocery shopping may be done at the local convenience store because of an inability to travel to the supermarket or to maneuver in a large store. Providing the names of grocery stores who deliver or those who have shoppers' helpers on staff may change the patient's diet and health.

Only when you have gained a thorough understanding of the patient's true needs can you be successful in improving his or her adjustment to visual loss. A good low vision clinic will address these social or rehabilitation concerns as well as optical needs. Asking appropriate questions will direct you toward success with the first aid chosen instead of trying magnifiers haphazardly. A patient who wants to see piano music will not benefit from a handheld magnifier. Both hands must be free to play the music. The same is true of those who love crossword puzzles. Hand magnifiers may be better than high-power spectacles, however, for reading recipes while cooking.

Questions to Narrow a Patient's Needs

Chief Complaint

What is the main problem you have related to your visual loss?

What visual struggle affects you the most in your daily life?

If we can restore one task for you with the help of aids, what do you most want it to be?

Vocational

What is your job?

What difficulties have you been experiencing in your work because of your eye problem?

What size print do you most often encounter in your work?

Do you have distance limitations such as working at a computer screen or a large drafting table? Have you measured this viewing distance?

General

Have you used magnifiers in the past? Were they helpful? Why or why not? How do you think we could improve on them for your use?

What kind of light do you use for reading?

What light is best for you?

Do you experience glare outdoors or difficulty adjusting to light changes?

Hobbies

Have you had to give up any hobbies or sports specifically because of your visual loss?

Does your vision prevent you from trying some sport or hobby you would like to try?

Activities of Daily Living

How do you shop for groceries? Can you see the labels and price tags?

Do you cook your own food? What is your biggest difficulty in preparing meals? Has your menu changed since your vision has become poorer?

Do you feel you can keep your house clean and finish the laundry or are you having trouble with household chores?

Can you read your own mail?

Do you write your own checks and balance your checkbook, or do you find it an impossible task?

Determine Level of Acceptance of Visual Loss

Sometimes patients receive low vision care too soon or at the request of a family member instead of from self-motivation. People come to ophthalmology exams with high expectations of cures and phobic fears of blindness. When presented with the news that nothing can be done medically, they may be overwhelmed with grief and fear. It will take some time for these strong reactions to evolve into a search for rehabilitation or an acceptance of the condition. The patient will forget anything you say about low vision or rehabilitation at the outset, and often will reject it. The time it takes a particular patient to accept the need for help will vary depending on personality, age, and family support.

Another common misinterpretation that a patient may bring to the low vision evaluation is a misunderstanding of his or her diagnosis and prognosis. Ophthalmologists like to cure blindness and perform surgery. They are not happy when there is no cure available, and sometimes unintentionally fail to discuss the subject with patients. If a patient is told to keep returning for follow-up, the impression may be that there will be some improvement or that a treatment is on the horizon.

What the Patient Needs to Know

- In this office we care about you.

- The questions you are being asked are not meant to be prying. We want to be aware of your difficulties so we can better serve you.

- We can show you optical devices to help with reading or distance vision. Your vision will not be as good as it used to be, but it can be better than it is at present.

- There are rehabilitation personnel readily available to help you with adjustment to both the physical and emotional difficulties of your visual loss.

There may also be a failure to understand the diagnosis itself because of lack of explanation. (If you discover that a patient has a poor understanding of his or her diagnosis and unrealistic expectations about the prognosis, you should inform the ophthalmologist or social worker involved so they can help the patient come to terms with the situation.)

During the low vision history, ask the patient (not a family member) to explain to you what is wrong with his or her eyes. Ask if the problem is expected to improve or worsen and what this means for his or her future. It is not the job of the assistant to provide the patient with the truth or discuss the prognosis, but the information will allow you to determine how much motivation the patient has to work with low vision aids (and their inherent problems.) If Mr. Jones thinks laser surgery is going to cure his eyes next month, he will not spend money on computerized optical devices. He also may not devote energy to practice reading at a very close reading distance. The well-informed patient who has accepted the visual loss is the patient who will be most successful with low vision aids.

Questions to Evaluate Acceptance

What medically is wrong with your eyes?
Is your vision going to get better? Worse?
Is your doctor still considering any treatments?
Do you feel that your vision problem has been thoroughly explained to you? Do you understand it?

Determine Level of Support of Family, Friends, and Agencies

A visually impaired person is disabled. Because a low vision exam is often the stepping stone to rehabilitation, it is important to assess the type of support your patient receives at home. Elderly low vision patients may not have a spouse or other family member who can drive or offer assistance in the normal activities of daily living. These patients, and those who live alone, will require more extensive help and referrals to social service agencies. Other seniors may live in an assisted-living facility and have most of these activities taken care of by the staff of the organization. They are luckier, and may do very nicely with just a magnifier and a subscription to a large-print newspaper. Be sure to contact the social worker at the assisted-living facility to help coordinate services.

A loss of sight robs a person of independence. Some dependencies are obvious, such as the inability to drive. There are other losses that are more subtle and personal, and can be even more devastating. As reading ability diminishes, private correspondence can no longer be private. A third person is necessary to read the mail. Personal financial records must be shared with others in order to write checks and balance accounts. This makes people feel very vulnerable. Because of these very personal needs it is vital that each low vision patient have the help of someone they can trust. If there is no family support or close friend, a social service agency or other professionals should become involved. A referral to a social worker is indicated.

If there is a good family network, write down the name and phone number of the relative who comes to the low vision evaluation. This person will be a good contact if any confusion arises. When training the patient in the use of low vision aids, ask one or more supportive family members to be present. Then if a problem arises at home, at least two people will be trained correctly, eliminating a need to call you for help.

Questions to Determine Support Level

Who brought you to the exam today? Are they friends or relatives?
Who do you call if you need help with shopping or other chores?
Do you have people whom you can trust and rely on for personal needs such as balancing your accounts?
Do you live with or near people who can help you? (Do not ask if he or she lives alone, for security reasons.)

Create Rapport and Win Trust

As you may realize by now, low vision is a very personal matter. It robs a patient of independence and dignity. There are many fears and frustrations involved. During past medical exams, however, doctors may have been businesslike, addressing only medical concerns. Patients learn to keep private matters to themselves. Although you seem interested, most patients will not divulge their personal fears or desires suddenly. They will explain gladly what they want to read, because they have been doing that since presbyopia affected them. It is socially acceptable to have difficulties reading the newspaper. The deeper concerns of patients may take a few visits to emerge, as you win their trust. By asking questions during the history, a dialogue occurs that will hopefully help the patient feel at ease and realize that personal issues are going to be addressed.

To help create this rapport as quickly as possible, educate your patients. Give a nonoptical aids catalogue to every low vision patient on the first visit. Talk about other people who have been helped in hobbies or vocations. Use anecdotes to explain what types of aids and agencies are available. A patient who does not know what is available will not understand how to seek help.

This may not sound like history taking, but is necessary for a successful low vision exam. Only after the patient is educated will he or she be able to give proper responses to questions regarding low vision history. On the other hand, it is important not to overeducate on the first visit. Patients who are nervous about visual loss are not going to retain very much information. For that reason, the history may evolve over the course of the exam or after several follow-up visits. Do not blindly stick to goals set at the outset, because the patient's needs and expectations may change as he or she realizes possibilities or experiences frustration.

To educate your patients, create a packet of information to present during the initial visit (Fig-

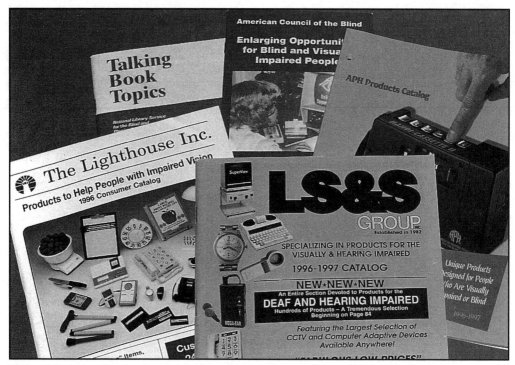

Figure 4-2. A sample of patient education materials that can be provided at the first visit.

ure 4-2). This will ensure that even if Mrs. Smith does not return for follow-up, information is in her possession to allow her to seek care on her own time. Such a packet might include:

- A list of local and national social service agencies offering help to visually impaired people. This may include optical help, social groups, support or advocacy organizations, banks that offer large-print checks to customers, and grocery stores that deliver or offer shopping assistance to disabled customers.
- A nonoptical aids catalogue such as that from The Lighthouse Incorporated or the National Association for the Visually Handicapped.
- A brochure from the American Academy of Ophthalmology or American Optometric Association about low vision care.
- A handout listing other publications that may be helpful to the patient such as information and an application form from the National Library Service for the Blind and Physically Handicapped and information from the National Association for the Visually Handicapped.
- A large print calling card listing the name of your clinic, the hours of operation, the person to contact with concerns or questions, and the phone number.

History Taking for the Pediatric Low Vision Patient

The low vision needs of children are different from those of adults. Many topics already discussed pertain to children, such as ocular and medical history, social support, and lack of independence. Family history of progressive diseases is very important also. That information will help determine the type of follow-up and social service intervention that may be necessary. The

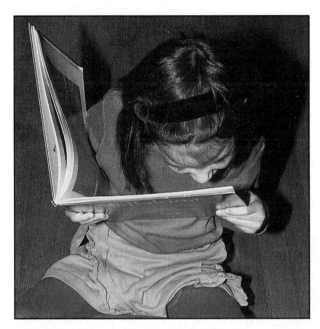

Figure 4-3. Children prefer to read at very close distances rather than use magnifiers.

real difference in the history of a child however, is in assessing the optical needs.

The major visual task of children is to see in school. Because of this, the teacher should be as involved in the low vision history as the parents. Teachers usually are willing to attend a low vision evaluation or at least to discuss the visual demands of their classroom over the phone. Teacher input is vitally important in deciding which aid to prescribe for a child. The parents alone usually are unaware of all the child's specific visual needs. A phone call to the school is done easily when scheduling a low vision appointment, and has great potential benefit.

Children have large reserves of accommodative ability, and can see print at near in spite of visual loss. They simply hold the material close and their accommodation acts as a built-in low vision aid (Figure 4-3). Although this eliminates the need for constant use of a magnifier for near, it should not preclude the prescription of one. Constant use of the full power of accommodation can fatigue the eyes, causing a lack of desire to read. A supplementary magnifier can help make reading more satisfying and comfortable.

Telescopes for distance viewing are good even for young children. They can be used in the classroom for board work, in the stands of a ball field to view sports, in auditoriums and movies to enjoy theater events, and in reading signs and bus route numbers to help with independent mobility. It is possible to prescribe telescopes at early ages including preschool and kindergarten. This gives the child an awareness of distance, and the telescope becomes a regular part of the viewing habits while there is no stigma involved. If presented with a telescope in the later grades, social pressure usually makes it difficult to accept.

Because children play hard it is imperative that they wear safety glasses. No matter what type of glasses are prescribed, the lenses should be polycarbonate and the frames should be sturdy enough to withstand strong forces. For sports with a potential for eye contact by a ball or racquet, frames should pass the American National Standards Institute (ANSI) Z-87 safety standards. For low vision children this cannot be emphasized enough. Children are more prone to accidents as a result of their visual disability, and have more to lose if they sustain further damage to their eyes.

Questions for the Pediatric Low Vision History

How far does the child sit from the board or other distant objects in the classroom (such as the clock)?

Is he or she able to read the appropriate size of printed material without much difficulty? What print size generally is used in his or her grade?

Is there a vision resource room or itinerant vision teacher available at the school?

Does he or she engage in any sports or extracurricular activities that require better vision? Has he or she wanted to participate in any of these activities, but felt limited visually?

How does he or she get to and from school? Can the child move freely about the school with out assistance?

How close does he or she hold material when reading?

What type of lighting is used for reading?

Are current glasses made with polycarbonate lenses? Even if there is no distance refractive error, are safety glasses worn?

Has a telescope or other magnifier ever been tried?

This discussion on history taking may sound involved, but it need not be tedious in actual practice. This thorough discussion is to help you understand why you are taking a history and some issues to consider. The actual questioning should only take several minutes. With practice you will become quite proficient at recognizing which questions to ask for a given situation. The following is a suggested form for taking a low vision history, to guide you in your investigation of each patient's needs.

OptT

Low Vision History

Date of visit:
Patient name:
Phone number: Age of patient:
Name and phone of support person (and teacher if applicable):

Ocular diagnosis:
Prognosis for vision:
Visual field loss:
Ocular history:
Medical history:
Current medications:
Allergies:
Patient's primary goal(s):
Distance needs:

Near needs:

Preferred lighting:

Magnifiers previously used and problems encountered:

Vocation:

Grade in school, name of school, name of teacher:

Hobbies:

Limited activities of daily living:
        Shopping/cooking:
        Grooming:
        Housekeeping:
        Correspondence/money management:

Method of travel/mobility:

Level of understanding of diagnosis/prognosis:

Living arrangements:

Wearing polycarbonate safety lenses?

Chapter 5

Assessment of Visual Function

KEY POINTS

- Move the test chart closer to allow the patient to experience success in reading more letters, and for a more precise evaluation of distance acuity. Record the actual testing distance.

- Always verify the refractometric measurement before beginning low vision testing. Optimal refractive correction is imperative.

- Near vision should be tested using continuous text cards and selecting the smallest size of print that can be read fluently.

Distance Acuity Testing

Traditional methods of testing acuity are not practical for low vision patients. Once acuity has dropped below 20/80 there are only a few letters per line on most distance test charts. They usually are variations of E, with one or two other easily memorized letters. This lack of choice causes inaccurate testing; recorded acuity reflects patient memory more than functional visual ability. Projected charts have the added problem of glare and can only be used in dim room light. Psychologically, if someone can only see the largest letters on a chart there may be a feeling of hopelessness and depression. Practically, if the patient only reads the big E, it does not allow the examiner to gain an accurate understanding of visual limitations and abilities.

Distance test charts designed for low vision alleviate these problems. Most of these charts are handheld rather than projected. They can be used in any lighting condition to better duplicate the normal situation of each patient. Most of the charts have optotypes that correspond to finer gradations of acuity between 20/80 and 20/800. For instance, there are letters that correlate to 20/120, 20/140, 20/160, and 20/180. Each line contains several characters so memorization is less likely.

Accurate acuity testing gives us the ability to assess magnification needs more clearly. For instance, a patient with 20/200 acuity needs 10 diopters (D) of magnification to read small print. Only 6 D are needed by the patient with 20/120 acuity. Using a traditional Snellen chart the acuity would be recorded as 20/200 and the magnification would be overprescribed, actually reducing the usable field of view. Patients also gain confidence when they can see many letters. They often remark that this is the first time in a long while that they can read the chart. This starts the low vision exam on a positive note, and encourages further success.

Handheld charts also allow accurate acuity testing situations when only "hand motions" or "counts fingers" has been recorded in the past. By moving the chart closer to the patient's eyes, the letter size can be doubled or quadrupled (Figure 5-1). Functional vision can be assessed even in the ranges of 20/3200 or greater.

Changing testing distances requires recalculation of acuity. On a chart designed for 20 ft testing distances, the optotype that corresponds to 20/200 acuity is 87 mm tall and subtends an angle of 50 min of arc on the retina. If the same 87 mm size object is moved forward to a distance of 10 ft, the testing distance is halved and the retinal image size is doubled. Record this acuity as 10/200 which is equivalent to 20/400 ([10/200] $\times$ [2/2] = 20/400). If the same size optotype is moved even closer, to a distance of 5 ft (¼ of 20 ft), record the acuity as 5/200 which is equivalent to 20/800 ([5/200] $\times$ [4/4] = 20/800). In this case the retinal image size is quadrupled.

Record acuity with the actual testing distance in the numerator and the optotype size in the denominator. Do not convert to "20" equivalents before recording. For example, if vision is tested at 5 ft and the 100-size letters are read clearly, vision is recorded as 5/100, not as 20/400. This allows future examiners to duplicate the same testing standards.

All patients should be examined first in daylight conditions. Ideally, also test office and retail workers under fluorescent lights. Specific lighting for other professions or avocations should be duplicated when possible to determine the patient's functional ability in his or her normal environment.

Contrast sensitivity and glare testing is indicated for low vision patients who have trouble with light changes. Patients with diabetic retinopathy are sensitive to bright light. Patients with retinitis pigmentosa cannot function well in low light, and experience delays in the ability to

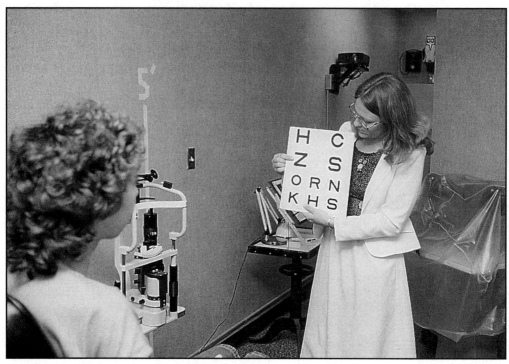

Figure 5-1. Acuity being tested with a handheld chart at a distance of 5 ft.

adapt from light to darkness. Patients may also have cataracts that have not been removed because of a poor visual prognosis. The glare associated with cataracts may exacerbate the vision loss from the underlying condition. Contrast sensitivity and glare testing will not diagnose these conditions, but can provide clues to functional problems. Counselling about lighting and absorptive filters can then be customized for patients' individual needs.

Verifying Refractive Error

Never assume that a patient is wearing his or her best refractive correction when arriving at a low vision exam. Frequently retinal surgeons have followed these patients for laser or other surgical treatments, and the health of the retina has been their priority. It may have been several years since the glasses were updated. In other cases, functional low vision problems may simply be overlooked refraction problems such as uncorrected high astigmatism. Each patient deserves thorough and accurate refractometry before low vision testing. This should be performed by the refractive expert in your office.

Low vision refractometric measurements are best performed "the old-fashioned way" with a trial frame and loose lenses (Figure 5-2). A refractor may be helpful during initial retinoscopy for convenience of the examiner, but the small visual apertures of the refractor limit the field of view. If a patient has central scotomas, the acuity will be better from a retinal point that is peripheral to the macula. The *eccentric view* and head position necessary to use this peripheral point will be impossible to achieve while using a refractor. Use a trial frame for refinement and vision evaluation. The best trial lenses to use for low vision are the full aperture lenses with a

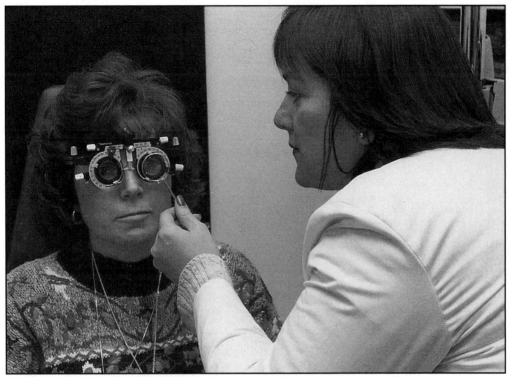

Figure 5-2. Refractometry using a trial frame and loose lenses.

thin metal carrier. The lenses with wide red or black edges provide very small visual apertures, especially in the higher powers, and are no improvement over the refractor. The chart should be held at a distance of 10 ft or even 5 ft, as in the initial acuity testing. Cylindrical correction should be determined with the use of a handheld Jackson cross cylinder as well.

Before refining cylinder or sphere it is necessary to detect the weakest lens that causes a noticeable difference in vision by the patient. Try +/- 0.50- and +/- 1.00-D lenses, increasing to +/- 2.00 D or higher as necessary until the patient is aware of a subjective decrease in visual resolution. This "just noticeable difference" will be the power of cross cylinder lens and spherical lens power used for refinement during refractometry. In addition, if a patient has a 0.50 D cylinder error, but his or her "just noticeable difference" is 1.50 D, the correction of astigmatism is not necessary. A spherical equivalent correction can be employed and the difference will not affect the functional visual ability.

Low vision refractometry is not routine, and some "tricks" may need to be attempted. A plano contact lens may be used for smoothing irregular corneal surfaces to provide the best refractive correction. The stenopaic slit and other "old-fashioned" devices may also prove helpful. Keratometry prior to refractometry may give clues about astigmatism. A refractometrist needs to be creative to find the optimum correction under less than optimum conditions.

Finally, remember that the measurement is being done at a distance closer than 20 ft. The final distance prescription will be focused for 5 ft or 10 ft (wherever the chart is being held). Remove up to 0.50 D of plus power to convert it to focus for optical infinity.

Near Vision Testing

Traditionally, ophthalmic and optometric assistants are taught to encourage patients to guess and struggle when testing acuity. Acuity is recorded as the absolute maximum number of letters that are guessed correctly. Because low vision is concerned with functional visual ability, the technique is different. If someone can identify individual letters of a given size, it does not necessarily correlate to reading ability. The size of print necessary for fluent reading is often considerably larger. In low vision, we record near acuity as the smallest size of print that can be read *fluently and easily*. When a patient begins to struggle with print, it is too small. Discontinue testing and record the previous, larger size print as the acuity level.

Perform near testing at two distances. First, allow the patient to read at his or her preferred distance. Measure and record the eye-to-print distance as well as the size of the print. This can be done with both eyes open. Allow the patient to use current reading glasses or magnifiers, remove distance correction, or use any other preferred method to see the near target. The goal here is to assess the current reading ability. Low vision aids that cannot improve on this level will not be accepted. No matter how scientific your measurements or logical your selection, an aid has to give the patient some functional advantage or it will not be used.

Second, measure the functional reading ability for each eye alone at a distance of 40 cm. This should be performed while the patient is corrected optically to emmetropia, and with an additional +2.50 add in the trial frame or attached to accurate distance spectacles with Halberg clips (Figure 5-3). This combination provides optimal focus without magnification at the 40-cm distance. This test will be used to calculate the power of magnification necessary for near tasks. Because improved visual function at near is the goal of most low vision aids, accuracy in testing is vital. The 40-cm distance must be kept constant and the optical correction must be optimum.

For both near testing situations, use reading cards specifically designed for low vision. These include paragraphs of continuous text instead of lines of isolated symbols. Generally, the reading cards are calibrated in meter equivalents (M units) instead of Jaeger or Point size. These M units were devised by Dr. Louise Sloan to simplify calculations of magnification.[1] Letters that subtend a 5′ angle on the retina when viewed at a distance of 1 meter are called 1M print. A 2M letter subtends the same 5′ retinal angle when viewed at a distance of 2 meters, 3M at 3 meters, etc.

This 5′ angle is the same size as that which projects on the retina from a "20" size letter on a Snellen chart at 20 ft. In terms of visual acuity, 1M at 1 meter and 20/20 are equivalent. The difference is that M units are calibrated in meters as is dioptric power. Because a 1-D lens has a focal length of 1 meter, there is a direct correlation between M units and diopters. This makes it easy to determine powers of magnification necessary for good reading ability.

Record near acuity as a fraction. The reading distance in centimeters is the numerator. The print size in M units is the denominator. For example, 40/4M means the patient can read 4M print

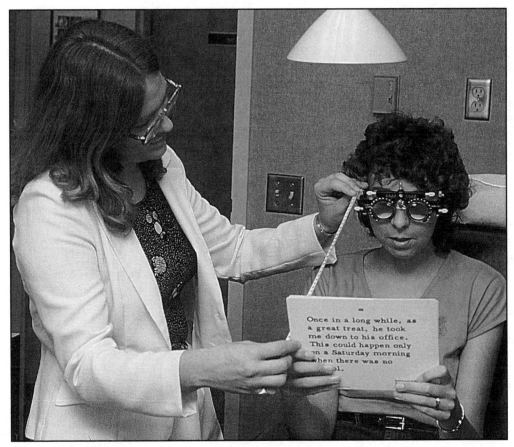

Figure 5-3. Acuity is tested at 40 cm with the best distance correction and a +2.50 add.

held at a distance of 40 cm. Remember to record the acuity where the reading is fluent, not where it is difficult.

In some cases there is a discrepancy of more than two M-units between the two eyes when tested at the same distance. In this case, the better seeing eye alone can be corrected by low vision aids. The power of the aid will be selected according to the acuity of this stronger eye. In high powers of magnification, patients use only one eye at a time anyway, so monocular correction will not be debilitating. If there is some interference from the eye with poorer vision, an occluder can be worn over that eye or the final near prescription can incorporate a frosted lens on that side. For temporary occlusion, dense Bangerter filters may be applied to the lens of the nonpreferred eye, and removed after the near task is completed.

Visual Fields and Low Vision

Visual field loss affects the functional ability of patients. Central scotomas can eliminate the ability to recognize faces, to read print, or to see straight ahead. To cope, the patient must adapt an eccentric viewing pattern and use magnification. Altitudinal defects from glaucoma or optic neuritis can make walking and reading very difficult. The patient may require mobility training and an eccentric viewing pattern. Hemianopic visual field defects render a patient vulnerable to dangers from objects on the blind side. Reading is very difficult when the visual field loss is left-sided because it is hard to find the beginning of the next line of print.

An interesting problem occurs when only a very small island of usable macular vision remains. In this case, patients do better with *lower* powers of magnification. Higher powers magnify images right out of the field of view and make reading much more difficult.

When providing low vision aids and making rehabilitation recommendations, the visual field loss should always be taken into account. If a patient does not have a recent visual field in the chart, fields should be assessed as part of the low vision protocol. This does not have to be sophisticated testing. We are not interested in the exact threshold sensitivity of every static point within the field of vision. We are only interested in scotomas or defects that impair function.

An Amsler grid test may suffice for patients with macular defects. A tangent screen is appropriate for those with hemianopic or altitudinal defects. At the very least, a confrontation visual field should be performed to detect gross loss of vision in large areas. A more accurate assessment from a Goldmann or automated perimeter is best. When testing, be sure to take the poor acuity into account. You may need to use a much larger size test object or move the patient closer to the test to gain an accurate result.

When referring patients for rehabilitation services, include a copy of the visual field with your referral. Visual fields are very helpful in deciding the course of training appropriate for each patient, particularly those with mobility issues.

Reference

1. Sloan LL, Brown DJ. Reading cards for selection of optical aids for the partially sighted. *Am J Ophthalmol.* 1963;55:1187-1199.

Bibliography

Corn A. *Foundations of Low Vision.* New York, NY: American Foundation for the Blind; 1996.

Step-by-Step Guide to Vision Assessment

1. Measure acuity monocularly at 10 ft or 5 ft with a handheld low vision distance test chart.

2. Record the vision appropriately to reflect the testing distance. For example, 50-size optotypes seen at 10 ft would be recorded as 10/50.

3. Measure near acuity with both eyes open in preferred conditions.

4. Verify refractive error using a trial frame and full field trial lenses, holding the chart at the same distance at which the acuity was recorded. Correct to infinity.

5. Remeasure distance acuity monocularly with the new optimum distance correction. This should still be done at 5 ft or 10 ft.

6. Put +2.50 lenses over the distance correction in the trial frame.

7. Hold a near-vision reading card at a distance of 40 cm and remeasure near reading ability with this combination of lenses. The reading card should have print in continuous text rather than as isolated symbols. Test monocularly for each eye. Record the size of type in M units as the denominator and 40 cm as the numerator. For example: The patient reads 4M print at 40 cm. Record as 40/4M.

8. Convert the reading ability in M units to a near acuity level. Do this by multiplying the M units by 100 to convert to centimeters. Divide the M units in centimeters by 40 to determine the power in diopters of the reading add that will most likely allow reading of 1M print. For example: Near vision is 4M.

   4M × 100 = 400 cm

   400 ÷ 40 = 10

   Use a 10 D reading add

9. Try the calculated power as a reading add in the trial frame if possible. The same power can be used to try a hand magnifier while the patient looks through his or her distance refractive correction. If a stand magnifier is tried, the magnifier power should be slightly higher and a standard reading add should be used along with it.

10. Perform contrast sensitivity, visual fields, or other testing as indicated before giving official trials with any aid or making final recommendations.

Chapter 6

Selecting Aids for Individuals

KEY POINTS

- Aid selection is determined by the patient's needs and goals as indicated by the history.

- The power of the near aid is determined by the patient's reading ability at a 40 cm testing distance.

- After several trials with a chosen aid, the final determination of whether it is appropriate and affordable will be made by the patient. Follow-up care is always necessary.

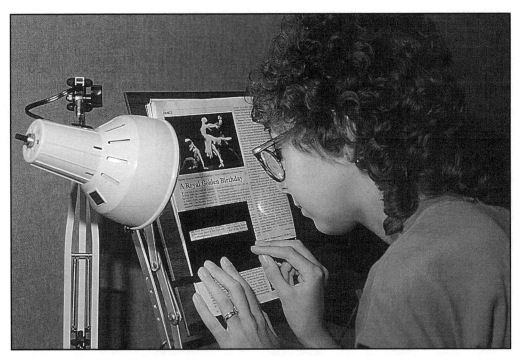

Figure 6-1. A typoscope helps isolate words on a page of print and reduce glare.

Among all the available optical and nonoptical low vision aids, a specific choice must be made for each patient. Some choices, such as the power and type of optical aid, are made by the primary low vision provider. Other decisions are made mainly by low vision assistants as they work with the patient in follow-up. As patients actually try specific magnifiers, they may decide that a particular model is completely unsatisfactory and a change needs to be made during training. Or it may become evident that a typoscope is necessary to isolate print while using a magnifier (Figure 6-1). For these reasons, low vision assistants should be intimately familiar with the steps to choosing aids and should also keep current with the whole range of nonoptical devices and rehabilitation services available.

Deciding on a Style

The first step in choosing an appropriate optical aid is to look at the patient's history. If someone has a task that requires both hands to be free, hand and stand magnifiers are essentially eliminated. Consideration should be limited to spectacles, loupes, and the few freestanding large field magnifiers. You should mentally narrow the choice of magnifiers for each goal of the patient. At the outset, introduce only one or two varieties that solve the most pressing needs of the individual.

For example, consider the case of a woman who loves to knit and do crossword puzzles but also needs to read her mail and recipes. She does not enjoy or desire long-term reading for pleasure. Spectacles, a magnifier on a neckstrap, or a freestanding magnifier would be the best choice for her hobbies because they allow freedom of movement for her hands (Figure 6-2). For mail and recipes, spectacles may be the best option, but a hand or stand magnifier can be considered as well. Spectacles for hobbies and a hand magnifier for mail are good starting choices.

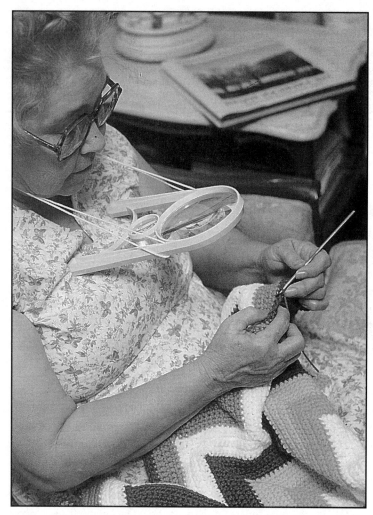

Figure 6-2. A magnifier on a neckstrap helps with crocheting.

Other case scenarios may indicate consideration of closed circuit televisions (CCTVs) and bioptic telemicroscopes. This would be especially true of individuals in college or in demanding professions. Severe visual impairment may lead you to suggest voice synthesizers and Braille. Each patient will be very unique.

Determining Power

Conversion of Reading Ability

The second step is to determine the power of magnification necessary for the patient. As discussed in Chapter 5, the method for testing low vision reading acuity is to test the patient's near acuity at a distance of 40 cm with a +2.50 reading add over accurate distance correction, and to record the smallest size of print that is read fluently. The vision is recorded in the chart as 40 cm over the M units. For example, if the best acuity is 5M, the vision is recorded as 40/5M. Once recorded in this manner, it is easy to put the information into practical use. The patient's reading ability in M units can be converted to dioptric equivalents for each task required.

Table 6-1
Lens Power/Acuity Chart
Near Acuity Tested at 40 cm

Size of Legible Print	Power of Lens to Try
1M	+2.50
2M	+5.00
3M	+7.50
4M	+10.00
5M	+12.50
7M	+17.50
10M	+25.00

Think of the notation 40/5M in terms of metric equivalents. The 40 was measured in centimeters, and the 5M refers to 5 meters. Convert the numerator and denominator into like terms (centimeters), so now the fraction becomes 40 cm over 500 cm. Divide the denominator by the numerator and it will give you the power of the first lens to try. In this case 500 ÷ 40 = 12.5, so the power of magnifier you will try first is 12.5 diopters (D) (Table 6-1). (Remember that with stand magnifiers, the power may have to be a bit higher, so start with a 15 D stand magnifier instead of 12.5.)

Providing 12.5 D in spectacles or hand magnifiers should enable this patient to read 1M print. Reading 1M print is considered a useful goal in low vision because it is similar in size to the average typeface in books, magazines, and most professional correspondence. Like the Snellen notation 20/20, however, it is only a standard. A patient may require stronger aids if he or she must read a smaller print size. Another alternative is to use a weaker aid and simply read larger print.

Note: A simpler way to determine power is to use the distance acuity, dividing the denominator by the numerator. For instance, a patient with 20/160 acuity would need an 8-D magnifier. (160 ÷ 20 = 8). This is very simple, and can be used in a pinch. Unfortunately, the distance acuity does not always correlate to near reading ability. If you learn the 40 cm test it will become just as easy to you, and will always be more reliable.

Age of Patient

At this point, the age of the patient is considered. If the patient is phakic and less than 30 years of age, he or she has between 9 D and 16 D of accommodative ability that can supplement the low vision aid power. Always subtract the patient's available accommodative reserve (one half of the total amplitude) from the calculated power requirement before selecting an aid. For example, a 6-year-old patient has 13 D of accommodative ability, so half of that, or 6.5 D, could be used for magnification without fatiguing the eyes. Instead of a 12.5-D magnifier, this child would only need a 6-D lens to read the same material (12.5 - 6.5 = 6). In fact, children often use their entire accommodative ability, holding material close to their eyes in lieu of using any near aid at all. Dividing reserves in half is more practical for those age 12 and older.

Refractive Error

The patient's refractive error must also be considered when deciding on a power. Patients with myopia have "built in" plus power and the amount of their refractive error can be subtracted from the power of the aid if it is going to be prescribed in spectacles or used without glasses. A patient with hyperopia needs the calculated power of the aid in addition to the extra plus needed to correct the refractive error. If a patient is going to be wearing glasses or contact lenses that fully correct the refractive error while using a magnifier, the power of the aid remains the same as the calculated power (12.5 D in our example).

Determining Focal Distance

Once appropriate lens power has been determined, calculate the focal distance of that lens. Divide 100 cm by the dioptric power of the lens to get focal length. In our example from the last section, divide 100 by 12.5. The focal length is 8 cm. *This focal length does not change if the power of the lens is increased or decreased to incorporate refractive correction of the patient, or to allow for accommodation.* This focal distance will determine the lens-to-print distance that will be necessary for optimum use of any hand magnifier or reading spectacles. A hand magnifier will be held above the page at a distance equal to the focal distance. Reading material will be held away from the eyes at a distance equal to the focal distance when low vision spectacles are worn.

Patient Input

Trials in the Office

After an optical low vision aid has been chosen using mathematics and the best experienced opinion of a low vision provider, it still may not be acceptable to the patient. A trial in the office is necessary to help the patient learn to use it correctly. In the office, conditions should be ideal. Use a reading stand to hold the book or magazine in place and at the proper angle. Appropriate lighting must be in place, and the reading material should be high contrast 1M-size print. A comfortable chair (without wheels) should be provided so that the only concern of the patient is the use of the optical aid. Instruct your patient on how to hold the lens, and where to position it in relation to the eyes and reading material (focal distance). It is important to meet with success at the outset to avoid unnecessary frustration.

Once your patient learns how to use the optical aid he or she should be left to try it alone for a few minutes. Provide ample reading materials including large- and small-print books, newspapers (including the obituary page and crossword puzzle), and typed correspondence (junk mail will do). After this practice session, your patient will either be happy with the lens and willing to try it at home, or will have reservations.

The patient's concerns may center on difficulty with field of view or maintaining focal distance. In these cases a little explanation and encouragement will help. However, if the magnification is inadequate or adjustment is very poor, try an alternative low vision aid. While working one-on-one you will become more aware of what the patient desires and how you might improve the situation. You will also discover if the patient is willing to adapt to new situations or is unable to cope with the inherent limitations of magnifiers. This should give you a clue as to how many different aids to try, and how much encouragement is needed.

One word of advice: Don't mistake a negative first reaction as failure. This is a new and difficult situation, and not necessarily what this person anticipated when coming for a low vision evaluation. Some people complain a lot, but adapt well to magnifier use with positive encouragement. Don't make rash decisions on changing aids until the patient has had time to try it at home.

Trials at Home

When one or two aids are identified as acceptable under the ideal circumstances you have created in the office, it is time to send the patient home. Keep a stock of aids to lend for home trial, and send most patients home with a magnifier or spectacles in hand on the very first visit. Instruct the patient and an accompanying family member carefully on proper lighting and remind them of the correct focal distance. A written reminder is helpful, because heads are full of new information after an initial low vision exam. It is easiest to keep preprinted pads on hand describing proper lighting and proper use of each major type of aid. Your handout should include several clear and concise steps such as the following, which relates to spectacles.

How to Use Your Low Vision Spectacles

- Always maintain a constant distance from your eyes to the paper. For your glasses, this distance is _____ inches.

- A reading stand will help you hold the book at a higher level than your tabletop.

- If the print goes out of focus, bring your face close to the reading material, then back away slowly until the image is clear.

- Always store the glasses in the case provided, as the lenses can become scratched easily. Clean the lenses only with lens cleaner and a soft cloth. Do not rub the lenses with dry papers or cloth.

A similar sheet of instructions can be provided for hand magnifiers, stand magnifiers, and telescopes as well as lighting. You can be as specific as you wish.

With instructions in hand, patients should be assigned a 1- or 2-week trial in their home or work environment. Actual "homework" assignments should be given to try during the 2 weeks at home. Instruct the patient to try their aid in and out of their own home with various lighting conditions. Be prepared for some phone calls during this period as patients experience difficulty. Frequently they are unable to function in their home environment as well as they did in the office. Home lighting is worse, and reading stands are probably not available to hold the material at the proper distance. Motivation may also decline as frustration develops and the reality of using the aids daily sinks in.

Follow-Up and Training

The first follow-up visit is generally very productive. Patients are much more able to discuss the advantages and disadvantages of their low vision aid, and speak more clearly about specific needs. At this time, power adjustments can be made if print size is still difficult to see. Individuals might tell you spectacles were ideal for home use, but were impossible at the grocery store. A pocket hand magnifier can be recommended.

What the Patient Needs to Know

- Medicare does not pay for low vision aids. Payment for glasses, magnifiers, and nonoptical aids is the patient's responsibility.

- There are agencies who might help you with payment if cost is a prohibitive factor to receiving the aids you need.

- Our office will work with you to try to set up a payment plan or to find alternative methods of payment.

A woman who plays bridge may complain that spectacles were fine for seeing cards in her own hand, but she was unable to see those on the table. Try half-eye instead of full-frame spectacles so she can look over them, and recommend large print playing cards. You can also instruct her to ask her partners to say aloud which card is being played.

Another patient may complain that looking up telephone numbers in the directory was difficult. Suggest a small stand magnifier of higher power, placed permanently on the telephone table.

Discuss lighting and reading stands more fully at this time. Also introduce the other nonoptical aids that would be most helpful. It is much easier to make suggestions based on very concrete desires. Several such needs will probably be identified at this visit.

Financial Considerations

Low vision examinations are sometimes covered by insurance, but third-party payers rarely cover the optical aids themselves. Medicare does not cover any low vision aids.

The cost of each low vision aid must be taken into account when recommending it, particularly to patients on fixed incomes. Low power, basic models of optical aids are relatively inexpensive. As of this printing, stock spectacles can range from $38 to $180 with increased cost relating to increased power. Hand and stand magnifiers range from $1.50 for folding pocket models to $150 for lighted stand varieties in attractive designs. Low power monocular handheld telescopes cost approximately $26 to $60, while bioptic telescopes can run in the $200 to $1000 range. CCTVs and other electronic appliances can cost more than $2,500.

Be honest with your patients as to the true cost of the devices you recommend. Become familiar with the cost, including your office's markup, so you do not quote the wholesale price from a catalogue to a patient. Cost is one consideration where patient input is mandatory.

There are a few ways to help your patients with the financial demands:

- The Veterans Administration will pay for low vision aids for veterans with service-related disabilities.
- Public schools are mandated to provide services to visually impaired students, and will usually pay for low vision aids within budget constraints.
- Young-adult through middle-age patients can receive monetary help from state vocational service agencies or services from the blind if the need for low vision aids is vocational in nature.
- The Lions Club civic organization devotes their philanthropic activities to assisting the needs of the blind. Local chapters are often willing to purchase low vision aids for

patients who are unable to pay.

- Elder care services, senior centers, and public libraries can be contacted to purchase aids for individuals in the community. These organizations usually purchase a few aids for community use rather than funding individual patients.
- Contact a local civic or school organization to have a "magnifier drive." Older people and their estates frequently donate glasses to the Lions Club, while useful magnifiers are thrown out. If you create a place to donate these items, it could be a good resource for "recycling" aids for use by patients in need.

Step-by-Step Guide to Selecting an Aid

1. Consider the primary goal of the patient. Must the hands be kept free?
2. Convert the near reading ability from M units to diopters to determine power, adjusting to allow for refractive error or accommodative ability if indicated.
3. Determine the focal distance of the chosen magnifier considering the power before adjustments were made.
4. Teach the patient to hold the magnifier or reading material at the proper focal distance. Use a reading stand, optimum lighting, and the desired size of printed material.
5. Allow the patient to try it while left alone for a few minutes with other sizes and choices of printed material on hand.
6. Make adjustments in power or style as necessary, considering the patient's financial situation when making decisions.
7. Send the patient home for 1 to 2 weeks to try the selected aid in the home setting. Supply the patient with a trial aid from your loan library as well as preprinted instructions on how to correctly use the aid. If possible, provide the information to a family member as well.
8. On follow-up, listen carefully to the patient's difficulties and successes, making adjustments or recommending additional aids as necessary.

Chapter 7

Rehabilitation and Referrals

KEY POINTS

- State-run and private agencies are available to help your patients. Check with your state government for local details.

- Professionals who provide assistance to blind or low vision patients include: rehabilitation teachers, rehabilitation counsellors, teachers of the visually impaired, orientation and mobility specialists, and occupational therapists.

Agencies and Professionals Who
Help People Adjust to Vision Loss

Agencies for the blind have been operating in the United States for generations. Blindness was one of the first disabilities to be recognized and adopted by philanthropic organizations. Because of this there are hundreds of agencies, organizations, self-help and advocacy groups available to your patients. The following is a general overview to make you aware of the various types of organizations available. A brief synopsis of the professionals who work with visually impaired patients is also provided.

Agencies

State Agencies

All states have an office that oversees support of blind and low vision individuals. Sometimes it is a separate agency specifically devoted to blindness, such as the Commission for the Blind in Massachusetts. Sometimes it is a division of another agency such as education; vocational services; or health, education, and welfare. Sometimes the support is splintered between several agencies. For instance, the department of education may handle children, vocational services may handle adults, and welfare may handle senior citizens, each within a separate subdivision of blind services. However they are organized, these agencies coordinate rehabilitation centers, public school assistance, and residential schools for the blind. They also provide monetary and vocational support to blind individuals.

Most states offer services to patients with low vision individuals as well as the totally blind, but often have some restriction based on acuity level and age. Some people may only be able to receive services if their vision loss falls into the category of legal blindness. Exceptions are usually made for those who have a poor prognosis, for children in public schools, or for those whose disability results in a loss of vocation. Services offered vary widely from state to state, so contact your state government for details.

Advocacy and Support Groups

There is a support group for almost all visual impairments and concerns. Specifically for children, the Hadley School offers free courses by home-study on issues related to parents and children with visual impairments.

The Hadley School for the Blind
700 Elm Street
Winnetka, IL 60093
1-800-323-4238

The National Association for Parents of the Visually Impaired (NAPVI) is a national organization for parents with visually impaired children. They have an information exchange for parents and can put parents of children with similar disabilities in contact with one another. They publish a quarterly newsletter that updates parents on social, medical, and educational resources for their children. NAPVI is also a clearinghouse on information about rare eye disorders.

NAPVI
PO Box 317
Watertown, MA 02272
1-800-562-6265

Similar groups for adults, which also engage in lobbying for blindness issues, are the National Federation of the Blind and the American Council of the Blind (ACB). The ACB also sponsors special interest affiliate groups such as the Visually Impaired Veterans of America and the Library Users of America.

ACB
Suite 720
1155 15th Street NW
Washington DC 20005
1-800-424-8666

The Council of Citizens with Low Vision and The National Association for the Visually Handicapped (NAVH) provide information and advocacy specifically to low vision individuals (instead of the blind). NAVH publishes newsletters called "In Focus" for youth and "Seeing Clearly" for adults. The NAVH also houses a 6,500 volume loan library of large-print books that can be borrowed by mail.

NAVH
22 West 21st Street
New York, NY 10010
1-212-889-3141

The Council of Citizens with Low Vision International
1-800-733-2258

The American Foundation offers a multitude of services and information to blind and low vision individuals as well as low vision providers. They provide information on most topics and publish pamphlets, books, and journals related to blindness issues. They also can be contacted for information on referrals and state regulations nationwide. The Lighthouse Incorporated offers low vision training to professionals, markets low vision aids, and provides medical and rehabilitation services to blind and low vision clients.

American Foundation for the Blind
11 Penn Plaza Suite 300
New York, NY 10001
1-800-232-5463
1-212-502-7600
Fax: 1-212-502-7777

The Lighthouse Incorporated
111 E 59th Street
New York, NY 10022
1-800-334-5497
Fax: 1-212-821-9707

The National Library Service for the Blind and Physically Handicapped (NLS) is a branch of the Library of Congress that has a lending library of recorded and Braille materials which, along with special cassette players or phonographs, are lent through postage-free mail. The NLS (see page 34 for address) has a special application form that includes a section to be completed by an ophthalmologist or optometrist. Copies of this application should be on hand in your office.

People who work with blind individuals may join the Association for Education and Rehabilitation of the Blind and Visually Impaired. Visually impaired workers themselves can belong to organizations such as the National Association of Blind Teachers, the American Blind Lawyers Association or the Visually Impaired Information Specialists, Incorporated.

Association for Education and Rehabilitation of the Blind and Visually Impaired
4600 Duke Street #430
POB 22397
Alexandria, VA 22304
1-703-823-9690

There are recreational groups such as Blind Outdoor Leisure Development (BOLD Incorporated [Aspen, Colo]), and Ski for Light International (Minneapolis, Minn) that coordinate camping and skiing trips for visually impaired children and adults. There is a Blind Golfers Association, the American Council of the Blind Radio Amateurs, and Friends-in-Art for poorly sighted artists and art lovers.

Support groups for various diagnoses include the Helen Keller National Center for Deaf-Blind Youth and Adults, the Retinitis Pigmentosa Foundation, The National Organization on Albinism, and the American Diabetes Association, among others.

Addresses

This is only a partial list of the numerous and diverse organizations that can be valuable resources for you and your patients. In lieu of listing individual addresses of each agency discussed in this chapter, the following resources can be used. Each of these directories is published annually and includes lists of many agencies that you can then contact individually:

"Directory of Agencies Serving the Blind and Visually Handicapped in the US"
American Foundation for the Blind (see page 80 for address)

"VISION Resource List"
Vision Foundation, Incorporated
818 Mt. Auburn Street
Watertown, MA 02172
1-617-926-4232
Fax: 1-617-926-1412

What the Patient Needs to Know

- Rehabilitation teachers will teach you methods to perform tasks of daily living.

- Rehabilitation counsellors can provide you with options for vocational training and advise you on where to receive help.

- Teachers of the visually impaired work closely with children in public schools to make sure their educational and rehabilitation needs are being met.

- Orientation and mobility specialists will teach you to travel independently in your home or in public places.

- Occupational therapists working in clinics can teach you to use low vision aids or other appliances efficiently, and to perform other tasks of daily living.

Rehabilitation Personnel

 ### Rehabilitation Counsellors

Rehabilitation counsellors are professionals who provide vocational assistance and information to blind and low vision clients. They develop and maintain files on each individual in their caseload and coordinate services provided by various organizations. Primarily hired by state agencies or rehabilitation centers, these individuals are similar to school counsellors. They provide information and referrals. They can also act as social workers, dealing with the adjustment and concerns of the blind client and family members. They frequently advocate for their clients in obtaining services from educational or vocational institutions. They also coordinate monetary support from federal agencies to fund the needs of clients. Rehabilitation counsellors are a good contact for low vision clinics, as they are usually aware of the resources available for each patient.

Rehabilitation Teachers

Rehabilitation teachers are more specific therapists. They work in rehabilitation centers, residential schools for the blind, and large public schools. They may also work on an itinerant basis travelling to public schools in less populated areas, to the workplace, or to the client's home to provide individual instruction.

Activities of rehabilitation teachers may include helping an elderly person organize kitchen cabinets by labelling each shelf front with a Braille or large-print sticker. They may teach Braille. They work with low vision patients in their homes, helping with the use of a magnifier or providing nonoptical aids. They help arrange the workplace in a useful manner for easier use by someone with low vision (Figure 7-1). Rehabilitation teachers work in a very hands-on manner and are a helpful resource for low vision clinics, as they can provide follow-up training after patients leave your office. If you are fortunate enough to work closely with a rehabilitation teacher, you can provide detailed instructions that can be invaluable to your patient's success with low vision aids.

Orientation and Mobility Instructors (Peripatologists)

Orientation and mobility (O & M) instructors are the professionals responsible for teaching clients to move around in their environment in spite of limited vision. They work in residential

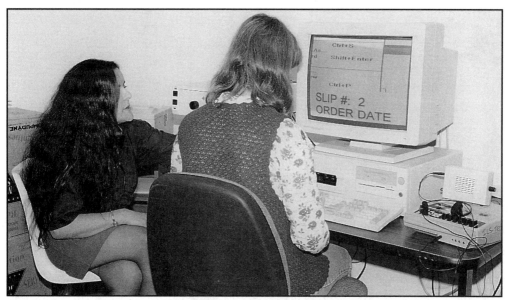

Figure 7-1. A rehabilitation teacher works with a client on computer skills.

centers, rehabilitation centers, and schools on a full-time or itinerant basis.

O & M instructors teach clients to become oriented to their surroundings by paying attention to sounds, landmarks, and clues. They teach clients to maneuver in their home setting by using self-protective techniques and arranging furniture and supplies in an organized manner. Orientation to the school or workplace is provided, and they also explain the logical arrangement of address numbering systems and street grids, enabling clients to use public transportation and find their own way in any private or public environment.

White Cane Travel

The use of white canes is taught by O & M instructors during the course of mobility training (Figure 7-2). These canes are used as extensions of the person's arm and provide tactile feedback about terrain. They give warnings about curbs, stairs, or other objects in the path that will be encountered or should be avoided.

Guide Dogs

Guide dogs are another form of mobility "device" that function much like a white cane. These dogs are trained to warn their master of any object in, or heading toward, their path that should be avoided (Figure 7-3). Besides the fact that they can be great companions, dogs are better than canes in several ways. They can give warning of dangerous objects at head level or of dangerous traffic patterns. The eyes of the dog take in a great deal of its surroundings, whereas a cane can only give feedback from the chest level down and only one or two steps ahead.

Guide dogs are not for every individual, however. The blind person must be in good physical condition. The master must be fast enough to keep up with the pace of a healthy dog, and strong enough to control the animal. Guide dogs can become lazy if they do not work daily, so the person who uses one must have a daily routine that takes them both out walking. Re-evaluation and retraining of dogs is necessary from time to time. (Note: It is incorrect to refer to guide dogs as "seeing eye dogs." The Seeing Eye is one guide dog center in New Jersey that is very well known. There are, however, many other centers that provide excellent guide dogs for the blind. The appropriate term to use is "guide dog.")

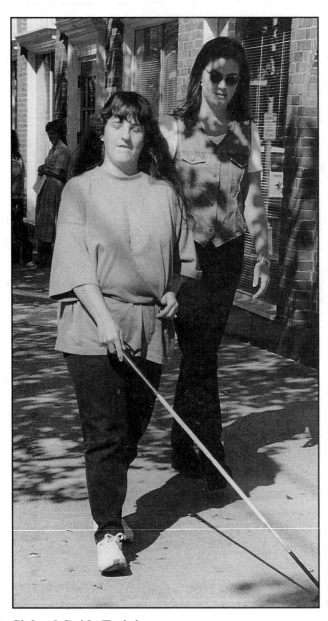

Figure 7-2. An orientation and mobility instructor teaches white cane travel.

OphA Sighted Guide Training

Orientation and mobility instructors also teach clients a technique known as "sighted-guide travel." This is when a blind or partially sighted individual holds onto the arm of a sighted person who guides them in unfamiliar surroundings. There will be many instances when a low vision provider will have to function as a sighted guide in the office, clinic, or hospital, so some of the rules are important to know.

- When guiding a blind person, always make contact first by touching the back of their hand with the back of yours, and stating that you will be happy to guide them to their destination (Figure 7-4). This allows them to locate you and place their hand in the correct position on your arm. They will grasp your arm from behind and slightly above the elbow (Figure 7-5). You can offer more support to elderly or unsure individuals if nec-

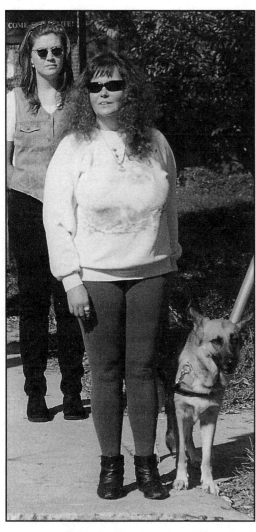

Figure 7-3. A guide dog is aware of dangers that a cane cannot detect, and is an excellent companion.

essary by allowing them to lean on your bent arm. (If your contact is rejected, allow the patient to walk on their own. Some people do not like to be guided.)

- Always allow them to hold your arm and walk a half pace behind you. Never guide them in front of you. You must walk ahead and be the leader, giving clues by your body movements as to when to start, stop, slow down, or turn.

- If you must step up or down stairs, stop completely on the landing and tell the person you are guiding that there are stairs. Allow them to hold the handrail with their free hand, maintaining contact with your arm. Begin to ascend or descend the stairs at a slow but regular pace. Do not pause until you reach the end of the staircase, but stop fully on the final landing to let the person know that you have reached the end. Allow them to catch up to you completely before proceeding.

- If you come to a doorway, open the door yourself, but allow the person you are guiding to close it behind you.

- When seating the person you are guiding, stop fully and remove his or her hand from your arm. Place that hand on the seat of the chair, and explain that he or she should take a seat. If there is a footrest in the way, either remove it or explain that it is there.

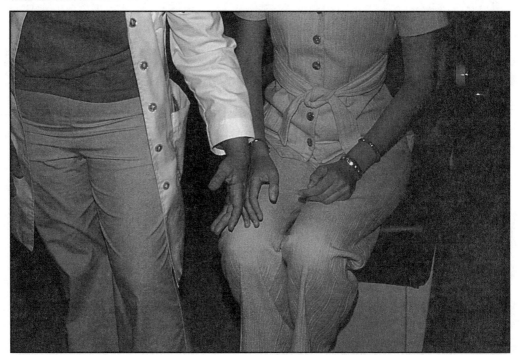

Figure 7-4. Touch the back of your hand to the back of the patient's hand. This allows the patient the option of taking your arm or not.

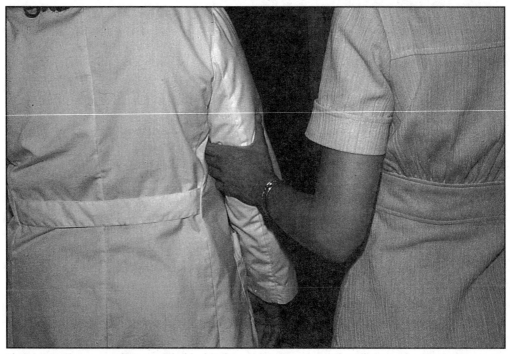

Figure 7-5. The person being guided holds the guide's arm above the elbow and walks half a pace behind.

If you follow these basic sighted-guide procedures, your patients will feel more comfortable. They will trust you more, and feel like a responsible member of the team as they close doors and hold handrails themselves. Even those who have not yet undergone training will feel more comfortable from the nonverbal and verbal clues you give, and from the confident manner in which you lead them.

Teachers of the Visually Impaired

Blind and low vision students have several choices of educational institutions. There are many residential schools for the blind where educational pursuits and rehabilitation are undertaken at the same center. The students live and study with other blind children. In 1976 a federal mandate, Public Law 94-142, was passed that required public schools to provide services to all handicapped children. Since that time most residential schools have only the most severely handicapped students in residence, and provide medical services as well. Since 1993, the Americans with Disabilities Act also mandated that public institutions make adaptations for persons with disabilities. This provides for a great deal of services to visually impaired students in the public schools, especially if the parents advocate for their child.

The majority of low vision and blind children attend public schools in regular classrooms. They sit close to the front of the class and use telescopes and low vision aids to help them see. Teachers of the visually impaired are trained to deal with the special needs of these students, and meet with them on a daily basis or as needed. Sometimes the teachers are itinerant, only coming to the school on a prescribed schedule. Other schools have resource rooms. These are special rooms where the student can come on a scheduled visit or just drop in. There are usually adaptive devices available in resource rooms such as closed circuit televisions and recorded material. Vision teachers will transfer handouts, reading assignments, and tests to large-print or recorded tapes.

One advantage of teachers of the visually impaired is that there usually is only one or two in a district. As a result, they will work with the child throughout his or her entire school career. The teachers provide continuity and a strong support to the child and the family. They will recommend low vision testing and work closely with parents, doctors, and low vision clinics to provide complete services to their students, and are intimately familiar with many helpful resources.

Occupational Therapists

Occupational therapists are medical professionals who help patients adjust to any disability in order to continue performing activities of daily living and/or vocational pursuits. They may work in hospitals, clinics, rehabilitation centers, or schools. Some low vision clinics have come to prefer the services of occupational therapists over those of rehabilitation teachers or O & M instructors because third-party payers pay for their services. The responsibilities of these professionals overlap a great deal, and one or all may be appropriate for your patients.

To contact rehabilitation personnel in your area, ask the state department of blindness services. Vision teachers can be located through the superintendent of schools.

Chapter 8

Setting Up a Low Vision Service

KEY POINTS

- It is relatively inexpensive to purchase the equipment needed to set up a low vision service, and the space it requires is minimal.

- Rehabilitation and referral agencies should be contacted before seeing your first patient so you have the necessary information on hand.

With proper equipment and space, it is possible to take care of low vision patients in any office or clinic. All that is required is a table that can accommodate a reading stand and light, reading materials, and a stock of low vision aids (Figure 8-1). The examination equipment is already available in most offices, with the exception of handheld distance test charts and near vision reading cards. Time is also required on the part of the low vision providers and assistants to compile a selection of referral materials. You must also decide what level of care your office intends to provide. The following discussion will provide the information you need to get started, no matter how involved you plan to become in low vision.

Equipment

Most offices set up a low vision service by first ordering a stock of aids and supplies. There are so many catalogs of aids available that it can become a considerable chore trying to decide which ones to purchase as the office stock. Each experienced low vision provider has his or her own favorites to recommend, and there are several individuals or companies who market their own starter kits complete with a storage cabinet. Of those, the one that is most complete is the Jose Low Vision Starter Kit® (Mattingly, Inc, Escondido, Calif). It includes all the basic aids and a good selection of nonoptical aids.

If your office cannot afford the $995 price for a complete starter kit, you can order aids individually or try one of the less complete and less expensive starter kits. The following is a list of the aids your patients will find most helpful.
- Several folding pocket magnifiers of 10 to 20 diopters (D)
- Handheld magnifiers of 5, 10, 15, and 20 D
- Stand magnifiers of 10, 15, 20, and 25 D
- Half eye prismatic spectacles of 6, 8, and 10 D
- Full-frame spectacles of 14, 18, and 24 D—Correction should be in both lenses so they can be tried by any patient, even though they will actually be used monocularly
- One or two monocular telescopes in 2.8× to 10× powers—The Selsi #162 monocular® is exceptionally versatile because it has interchangeable lenses for powers of 6× and 8× in one scope
- Several Solarshields® or NoIR sunglasses for glare control

You will also need a stock of nonoptical devices. At a minimum this should include:
- Check and writing stencils
- Telephone dials with large print
- Large-print syringes or syringe magnifiers for diabetics
- Needle threaders
- Some recreational materials such as large print playing cards and one or two games
- Several typoscopes for office use (while training with aids) and to lend

Examination materials that are necessary include:
- Distance charts
- Continuous Text Reading Cards
- Reading stand
- Appropriate lamp
- Reading materials

A good distance chart for adults is the *Low Vision Chart Set* (Goodlite, Inc) by Gerald Fonda, MD. These charts come in a set of two to help avoid memorization. They are simple to use, logically designed, and have helpful conversions for different testing distances.

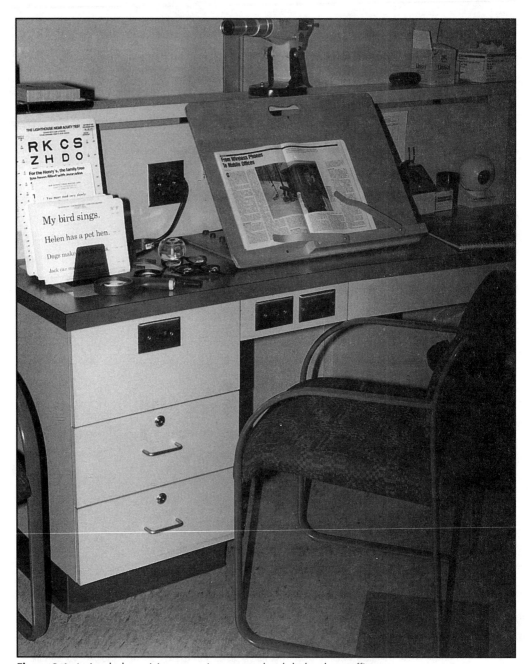

Figure 8-1. A simple low vision setup in a general ophthalmology office.

The HOTV distance test chart (Goodlite, Inc) is best for pediatric use (Figure 8-2). Children older than 4 or 5 can usually name the four letters that make up the chart. Younger children can use an accompanying card to match the letter at distance to the proper one on the card. This chart is much more accurate than the available handheld picture charts, and has more identifiable symbols. For near acuity testing, *Continuous Text Reading Cards* are necessary for both adults and children. For younger children who cannot yet read, an *HOTV near card* is excellent.

Your office will also need a *reading stand and appropriate lamp*. The light should be a good quality, flexible arm reading lamp with a heavy base so it will not fall over. It should have a metal

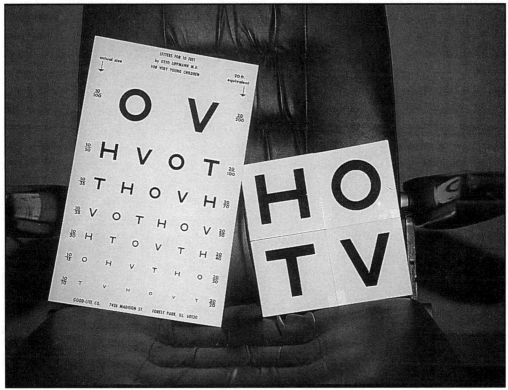

Figure 8-2. The HOTV test chart with a matching card for pediatric use.

reflective shade and a stock of 60-watt bulbs. Several types of *reading materials* should be within easy reach of the reading stand (Figure 8-3). These should include:

- A large-print book or *Reader's Digest*®
- *TIME*® or other news magazine
- Newspaper front page
- Newspaper obituary page
- A piece of correspondence such as a utility bill
- A Bible
- A supply of children's books and comics

Before seeing any patients, you should also compile the stationery and office supplies you will need. This includes:

- Large print calling cards with your clinic name and phone number
- Packets of informational materials to give to each patient (Chapter 4)
- Instructions for the use of each of the major types of aids: hand magnifiers, stand magnifiers, spectacles, and telescopes
- Catalogues from optical and nonoptical aid vendors
- Referral forms for rehabilitation agencies and the National Library Service for the Blind and Physically Handicapped

(The addresses for vendors of each of these supplies are listed in Chapters 2 and 3.)

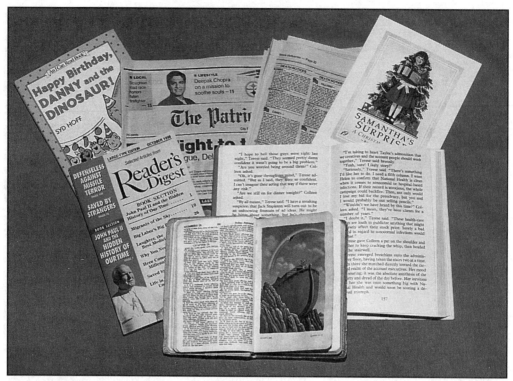

Figure 8-3. Reading material on hand should include a newspaper with obituary and stock market pages, a large-print book and/or magazine, children's reading material, and a Bible.

Finding Referral Agencies

Before seeing your first patient, locate your state agencies and familiarize yourself with the state laws governing care to the visually impaired. By contacting the state agency that oversees care to the blind, you will be directed to several other sources. Each one leads to many others in a pyramid fashion. On your first contact, ask about services for children as well as services for working adults and seniors. Find out the name of several low vision clinics and rehabilitation centers in your area and go visit them. Make an appointment with a rehabilitation counsellor to ask questions about state and federal help and regulations. For each contact, determine how to make referrals and request copies of all necessary forms.

Working With Low Vision Clinics in Your Area

If you only intend to offer minimal care to your patients, you have several options. The first is to provide written materials about low vision support agencies and make appropriate referrals only. These referrals would include the state agency that oversees low vision clients, any appropriate support organizations, and a separate local low vision clinic for evaluation and follow-up care. You should visit several low vision clinics ahead of time to determine which is best for your patients. Do not just refer to the local office that sends patients for surgery. Look for the low vision clinic that offers the best services and follow-up for your patients.

Another option is to evaluate low vision patients in your office, providing simple magnifiers and nonoptical aids. A referral to another low vision clinic can be made if the patient requires more sophisticated devices such as bioptics or closed circuit televisions. In this case, you must be more responsible for referring patients to appropriate agencies and rehabilitation personnel for continued care, as your office will be the primary contact for each of these agencies.

Involving the Community

There are many possibilities for low vision clinics to become vital players in the local community, bringing together diverse groups with interests in low vision. By inviting vision teachers to the evaluation of their students you will become involved in the schools. Libraries are always receptive to new materials and would appreciate information on where to send for books and periodicals pertaining to low vision. Civic organizations such as Lions Clubs like to have guest speakers, and those interested in eyecare are always welcome. A discussion of the services your low vision clinic provides will go a long way to bringing in more patients, and also perhaps some funding when needed.

If your clinic or office is in a small community, you may be the only resource for many people who have been looking for help. You can become a clearinghouse for information or even create a support group for local families who have a relative with low vision. In 1981, a local group evolved in Augusta, Georgia, from just such an effort. Local teachers, low vision providers, rehabilitation personnel, and families with low vision children began to meet monthly. The first half hour was spent mingling and talking and sharing stories. Then a speaker from an agency or organization would talk for a half hour, followed by refreshments and more mingling. It was sometimes difficult to get the families to leave because they shared so much in common and had been experiencing it alone for so long. It took very little effort on the part of the organizers, and brought together diverse parts of the community with common interests. Be creative in your own area and you never know what might evolve.

A simpler way to provide services to your patients is to organize a monthly meeting of patients with similar diagnoses. This can be in your office or in a public setting. There is no need for a specific group leader, although you may give a talk on the disease process and take questions. Mostly, it will be to allow time for patients with similar experiences to share time and stories with one another. The best support for someone in need is the companion of other people with a similar disadvantage. They support each other emotionally, and share information about agencies or supplies they have found to be helpful.

Coding and Pricing

Coding to bill for low vision services is a complicated process with few specific rules, and must be individualized in each office. It is illegal to "price fix," so many established clinics will be unwilling to offer you information about their specific billing practices and fees. Each office must tailor their own system based on their past practices. Remember that Medicare does not cover low vision aids at all. The payment for optical devices is up to the patient. For instructions and possible pricing for examinations and training, contact your local Medicare affiliate. Refer to your coding book for the following guidelines:

Diagnosis codes, from the American Medical Association ICD-9 Coding Directory, approved for use in low vision rehabilitation are currently between 369.01 and 369.76. The number varies depending on the acuity level of each eye. See your diagnosis coding directory for details, and watch for updates.

Chapter 9

The Psychology of Visual Loss

KEY POINTS

- People who experience loss of vision undergo a grieving period for the "death" of both their previous identity and their independence.

- When partial vision is lost, there is always a fear that total blindness will occur next.

- It is far better for eyecare professionals to be honest than to offer insincere encouragement about prognosis. We should educate and not avoid discussing the realities of visual loss.

Changes in Self-Image

Each time we see a patient who has a disease that leads to loss of vision, we must be aware of what that patient is experiencing at home. We see them when they come to our office, and we hear their answers to the questions we ask when taking the history. Usually the questions we ask are strictly medical: "Has there been any change?" "Have you been looking at your Amsler grid every day?" "Have you noted any new floaters?" The answers to these questions do not give us information about anything in which the patient is interested. Patients are worried that they are going to be totally blind. When we ask if patients have noted any changes, they hear "Has your vision gotten worse like I expect it is going to?" The patient has likely been losing sleep and crying to friends about the fear of blindness. If the vision is poor enough to limit activities of daily living, the patient is also undergoing loss of self-esteem and a multitude of other blows to his or her ego.

In his classic book, *Blindness: What It Is, What It Does, and How to Live With It*,[1] Reverend Thomas J. Carroll outlines twenty substantial losses, or "deaths" of previous characteristics of personal identity that people suffer when they lose their sight. Fourteen of these losses are also applicable to the patient with low vision. The severity of their impact is directly related to the type and severity of the visual loss. Reverend Carroll's list of losses includes:

1. Loss of Physical Integrity

When a person loses vision, it becomes difficult to be at peace with the identity of "self" that has been developed over a lifetime. He or she is no longer a whole person, but is a disabled person, with all the negative connotations that includes. The person begins to doubt his or her self-worth and ability to function or compete in "normal" society. There is also a terrible fear of imminent total blindness.

2. Loss of Confidence in the Remaining Senses

Many people believe that the remaining senses compensate by becoming more acute when a person is blind. This is not true. In addition, most of the low vision population consists of elderly people. These patients experience the same age-related loss of hearing, taste, and smell as their perfectly-sighted contemporaries. Sight is our most reliable sense, and is used throughout life to validate the input from the other senses. For instance, when we hear a sound we *glance* in the direction of its origin to verify that it is, in fact, the sound we thought. Without the ability to validate the other senses by visual verification, low vision patients become afraid of their own ability to make sensory judgments. Vision has always been automatically used as a "double check" to sensory inputs from taste, smell, and touch as well. Now the person must completely reorient himself or herself to other environmental clues.

3. Loss of Mobility

Mobility refers to our ability to move about our environment independently. With a loss of vision people become unable to drive, causing their world to shrink. Even if able to walk or use public transportation, they may be afraid to descend stairs for fear of falling. They may be afraid to use buses for fear of being stranded from inability to read the timetable or a clock. They become fearful of curbs and stones in the sidewalk, and are unable to read road-crossing signals. Significant loss of vision can make a person a captive in his or her own home.

4. Loss of Techniques of Daily Living

With poor vision it becomes very difficult to tell if your home or your person is dusty or soiled, and frequently leads to unwitting negligence of personal appearance. This can be a tremendous emotional strain to the self-image of the person who has always prided himself or herself on a neat appearance. Shaving, applying makeup, eating, cooking—each of these things that we take for granted becomes a challenge to the person who loses vision.

5. Loss of Ease of Written Communication

The loss of the ability to read brings with it an inability to read one's own mail, correspond with friends and businesses, and enjoy the daily paper. This is the only loss that is widely recognized, and frequently the only one addressed during a low vision evaluation. It is very important, and can usually be helped with low vision aids, but it is far from the only issue we should address.

6. Loss of Ease of Spoken Communication

In conversations we do more than hear the words of others. We watch their facial expressions and gestures for clues as to the humor or actual intentions of the words. Frequently we can tell more about a person from the look on his or her face than from the words that are spoken. With visual loss, people lose this important part of communication and are at the mercy of the words alone, leading to awkwardness in many social situations. Another aspect of this problem is being unable to recognize friends when passing them on the street or at social gatherings. A person who loses sight may now be perceived as being unfriendly by unwitting acquaintances. This is especially true for low vision patients who are able to function fairly normally and show no outward signs of their disability. Many relationships are lost as a result of this misunderstanding.

7. Loss of the Visual Perception of the Pleasurable

When sight is lost, frequently the most painful part is the inability to see the faces of loved ones. Also, other personally valuable objects such as pieces of jewelry or collections are no longer able to be enjoyed in quite the same way.

8. Loss of Recreation

Recreation includes anything done for pleasure such as sports, playing games, needlework, or going to movies. Many activities previously engaged in for the sheer enjoyment of it become difficult or impossible when vision is lost. Loss of relaxation and tensional outlets can be very detrimental to physical and emotional well-being.

9. Loss of Career, Vocational Goal, or Job Opportunity

This loss is the most severe to the person who loses vision in youth or middle age. When we lose our ability to function in our job we lose the identity that we have fashioned for ourselves over many years. Add to this the loss of income, and it can be a severe blow to self-esteem and lifestyle. Patients often feel useless and depressed.

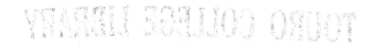

10. Loss of Financial Security

The loss of a job leads to lack of income at the same time that a loss of vision increases expenses. There are more doctor and pharmacy bills, more costs for transportation to appointments, and less insurance coverage. Other increased costs related to loss of vision include that of readers, delivery people, housekeepers, and other services that stem from an inability to perform tasks of daily living. Keep this financial hardship in mind when recommending expensive low vision aids.

11. Lack of Personal Independence

Each of the topics already covered speak of the painful loss of independence caused by losing vision. Added to this problem is that family members and friends like to have someone to "take care of" and may try to increase the patient's dependence rather than have them return to a level of independence. As Reverend Carroll so aptly states, "Death to independence means an end to adult living."[2]

12. Loss of Social Adequacy

This is the loss which is visited upon blind people by society. They are treated differently by the people around them. They are now pitied and are no longer "part of the group." A woman may now be referred to as "poor Mary" instead of just "Mary." This social separation is felt by the person with poor vision when he or she is treated differently by peers, social groups, and even family.

13. Loss of Self-Esteem

When a person has lost independence, career identity, financial security, sociability, and the basic trust of his or her senses, it is a terrible blow to self-esteem. His or her total sense of self has to be re-evaluated, and usually begins with an overwhelming sense of uselessness, inadequacy, and fear.

14. Loss of Total Personality Organization

There are many ways that people deal with these losses according to their own personality type. Some of the typical reactions are:
- Depression—Fear and an inability to cope lead to depression.
- Escape—Patients believe that the vision is going to improve, especially with trust in God. They may stubbornly continue to attempt some tasks (such as driving) even when they can no longer be done safely.
- Blame—Patients may blame all of their problems on the visual loss, or on other people. Every hardship in life will be seen as the result of someone else's carelessness.
- Escape into blindness—Patients give over to dependence and revel in it. These people become overly dependent and avoid all responsibility for their own needs.
- Hostility and resentment—Patients may harbor anger against all of society and its hardships, blaming it for all their suffering. These people may become chronic complainers about every little thing, when in fact it is the visual loss that is causing frustration and fear.
- Anxiety—The person who experiences severe anxiety attacks may have physical symptoms such as ulcers, high blood pressure, and sleeplessness.

What the Patient Needs to Know

- Adjusting to visual loss requires mourning the loss of your independence. It is normal to be sad, frightened, and depressed.

- There are other people experiencing the same difficulties as you. We can put you in touch with others who are sharing your same fears if you would like some peer support.

- There is hope. Other people have achieved great things in spite of total blindness. Although you will not be able to function as you did before, you can still function at a very high level.

Each of these blows to identity occur in each individual we see as low vision patients. The losses are manifested in differing ways and differing intensities, but the problems exist for every visually impaired person. When the visual loss occurs slowly over a long period of time, these problems may take a long time to work through. Some patients try so desperately to rely on their vision that they do not realize when it is time to relearn ways of doing things.

One low vision patient, an 18-year-old boy with glaucoma, had a binocular visual field that had deteriorated to only a 5° angle. When crossing streets he constantly looked down and hunched over, desperately seeking to see the curb and the crosswalk stripes on the road. Because he was so reliant on his vision and afraid of trusting his other senses he rarely walked alone. When he was finally sent for rehabilitation he learned to use a cane to seek the curbs, and he used his vision to look across the street for the crossing sign or traffic signal. He then was able to feel more confident, and use his vision more efficiently. He was able to walk upright and society began to accept him as more "normal." Just learning to reorder his way of doing things allowed him to regain his independence.

For other patients, if the visual loss is more sudden, the problems of dealing with it can be much more acute and result in near paralysis of ability to function for a while. These patients are not receptive to low vision aids until they have had time to work through their own emotional trauma.

Both types of patients need to let go of old habits and relearn new ways of doing things and new adaptive techniques. This comes easily to some, with difficulty to others, and to still others it is never possible. We must understand when we suggest low vision aids that the patient who is unsuccessful just may be unable to accept the necessity of the visual aid. Given time, that same person will be willing to admit that his or her vision is not going to improve and probably not going to decline further either. Only at that time will an aid be accepted. The same patient who was unsuccessful originally may be the most successful once the visual loss has been accepted.

Reactions of Families and Friends

Besides the personal problems the patient is experiencing because of the reorganization of his or her own self-image, there can be external problems. Families may have a very hard time accepting the difficulties of visual loss. Problems usually fall into two camps. First are the families who overreact and want to take care of the patient. These families are easy to spot. They always fuss over the patient as he or she walks into the room. They hold on to him or her until

What the Patient Needs to Know

- You are not stupid, you are only disabled.

- Other people will not understand your disability unless you inform them. They do not mean to be insensitive, they simply do not understand.

- When you become comfortable with your own visual loss and regain pride in yourself, you will be able to help others see your potential as well.

safely seated in the chair, jump up at any sign of need, and frequently speak for the patient as well. These families mean well, but can be a great hindrance to the patient's ability to regain his or her self-esteem, self-worth, and independence. If someone is taking care of all your needs, it is impossible to take responsibility for yourself.

The second difficult type of family is one steeped in denial. Low vision patients almost always look normal. They do not have any outward signs of their handicap, and nothing external has changed. Except for patients with debilitating visual field loss, patients can usually walk alone and take care of most of their own responsibilities. The family does not understand (and often does not believe) when Mother cannot shop alone or keep up with correspondence. The family members believe that she is just looking for sympathy or acting lazy when she asks for help or complains about her inability to function. This type of family can be very devastating, causing the patient to pretend to be much more self-sufficient than he or she really is. Long-term problems can result from mistakes in paying bills, accidents while cooking or attempting to drive, and the emotional inability to ask for help when it is needed.

This lack of awareness of visual loss is also manifested by friends and acquaintances. A low vision person can be perceived by friends as being suddenly clumsy or stupid. Others may doubt the visually impaired person's intelligence when they consistently play the wrong card or write down the wrong phone number. They are perceived as being unfriendly when in fact they cannot see the faces of people across the room. All of these misunderstandings can lead anyone to begin to decline social invitations, leading to loneliness and depression. Each of these problems can be exacerbated if the patient lets pride get in the way and does not explain to peers that he or she is experiencing a visual loss.

Reactions of Health Professionals

As health professionals we are also guilty of avoidance and denial. Often when dealing with low vision patients we tell them how well they are doing. We praise them for reading the 20/100 line this visit when last week they were only able to read 20/100-1. It is easy to say, "Oh, your vision is much better this time." Although innocently meant as encouragement, this type of behavior helps lead the patients to denial and false hope. They look to their eye appointments with great anticipation, and the comments of eyecare professionals become very important. If we tell patients they are doing better, they think they hear that their vision is going to improve and they are going to "get better." This type of false hope only leads to a delay in the patient's ability to accept the visual loss and seek help in dealing with it. This in turn stands in the way of regaining self-esteem and independence.

What the Patient Needs to Know

- Using your eyes will not harm them. Nothing you did in the past has caused you to lose your vision.

- Low vision is a term that means that your vision is poor. It does not mean that you are blind or that you will become blind.

- We in eyecare want to do everything we can to enable you to see well. Sometimes we can no longer make your vision better. But we can help you adjust to your new situation if you will work with us.

- If you misunderstand the meaning of your eye disease or are not sure what it means for your future, please ask. Although we understand your fears in general, we are not aware of specific concerns until you mention them.

What You Can Do to Help

 ### Honesty and Tact

When dealing with patients who are experiencing visual loss, realize that addressing the difficulties is not going to embarrass them. It may disappoint them, but like the firm discipline of a good parent, honesty is best. Eyecare professionals should talk to patients honestly and without pity or condescension. First and foremost, the diagnosis must be explained fully in laymen's terms. If the patient does not understand what is wrong with his or her eyes, fears and misunderstanding will result. The prognosis should be completely explained as well. If the vision is going to remain poor, it should be recognized as such. False encouragement should not be given. If the vision is 20/100 for several months, it is far better to let the patient know that you understand he or she must be experiencing difficulties in daily life. Ask what types of problems they are encountering and suggest some nonoptical aids that might help. This would also be a good time to offer a copy of a nonoptical aids catalogue, even before a formal low vision evaluation. During this explanation of visual loss, all patients must be reassured that the loss of vision is not due to any action on their own part. Most patients fear that they have done something in the past to harm their eyes such as read too much, sew too much, or watch television in the dark. Reassure each patient that using their eyes will not harm them. Otherwise, they might stop attempting to read or function visually.

Use the terminology the patient will need in the future. Discuss the idea of "low vision," and how it is different than blindness. Let the patient know that their vision is poor, but is not going to be completely lost. Also be honest that they are probably not going to note much improvement, either. Many patients are confused about the term "legal blindness." Educate each patient on the difference between low vision, legal blindness, and total blindness. Mention the existence of low vision services, and offer a referral when they feel ready. All of this can be done while still considering laser and other treatments as a means of educating the patient. It can be done tactfully and honestly.

Our own attitudes toward blindness and rehabilitation color our treatment of patients with poor vision. If we are afraid of blindness, we will be afraid to be encouraging. If we feel that rehabilitation is some type of nightmare to be avoided, we will not refer our patients properly. If we feel that blindness is a failure in the eyecare system, we will feel disillusioned and attempt to avoid dealing with the consequences.

The best way to overcome these false ideas is to visit a rehabilitation center for the blind. When eyecare professionals are educated in the possibilities open to partially sighted individuals they will feel more comfortable and make appropriate referrals. A visit to a local center for the blind is recommended for every person in eyecare, but most particularly to those who are setting up a low vision service.

Patients with severe loss of vision may not recognize who you are, or even when you enter or leave the room. If a patient cannot see your face, he or she is not sure if you are speaking to them or to someone else in the room. Always say the patient's name when addressing him or her, and introduce yourself in the same context. Physical contact, such as a touch of the shoulder or handshake are also reassuring and help the person know your proximity. This can be simply done as you call the patient in from the waiting room. "Hi Mr. Davis, I'm Linda, the low vision assistant. I'll walk with you to the exam room and we'll see how you are doing with your new glasses."

Support Groups

Loss of vision is very isolating, and each patient who experiences it feels alone and frightened. The ability to share the experience with others who are experiencing a similar loss is invaluable. You or your office can offer an extremely valuable service to your patients by facilitating a way for similar patients to meet. There are several ways this can be accomplished depending on the interest and enthusiasm of your office staff:

1. A bimonthly evening session can be offered in your office or at a local meeting hall. It can be a social gathering only if desired, with your office merely coordinating the place to meet and sending out flyers to the appropriate patients.
2. The sessions can be more formal, with a guest speaker and social hour each time. Guest speakers can be invited from local rehabilitation agencies, low vision aid vendors, low vision clinics, and other support or informational groups.
3. Patients can be given the name and phone number of other consenting patients so they can call one another with questions or support.
4. Patients with similar diagnoses and poor vision can be scheduled the same afternoon each month. Then the lunch hour can be set aside for them to meet one another if they want to come early to the appointment. (Many patients who need help with transportation come to visits early anyway.) This way, there would be something positive for them to do while they are waiting. One day per month could be "macular degeneration day," one day could be "diabetic retinopathy day," etc. That way the patients do not have to go to another site to make contact with one another.

Other ways of putting patients in contact with one another are as numerous as your imagination will allow. Providing patients with the opportunity to share experiences can only be helpful and ease them through their transition into a mentally healthy low vision person ready for low vision aids and rehabilitation. It is important, however, to try to arrange for patients in different stages of adjustment to attend these meetings. If all the patients have been recently diagnosed, they may only share their fears and resentments. People who have worked through their loss, adjusted to visual aids, and once again gained independence are important role models. They should be available to offer encouragement and hope for the future.

For children, and parents of blind children, this idea of group therapy is even more important.

Local chapters of the National Association for Parents of the Visually Impaired (NAPVI) are available around the country. By contacting the national branch in Watertown, Massachusetts, parents can get information and support from other parents. The address for NAPVI was given in Chapter 7.

References

1.Carroll T. *Blindness: What It Is, What It Does, and How to Live With It*. Boston, Mass: Little, Brown & Co; 1961.

2.ibid., pg 68.

Bibliography

Carroll T. *Blindness: What It Is, What It Does, and How to Live With It*. Boston, Mass: Little, Brown & Co; 1961.

Dickman I. *What Can We Do About Limited Vision?* New York, NY: Public Affairs Pamphlet; 1977.

Emerson D. Facing Loss of Vision: The Responses of Adults to Visual Impairment. *The Journal of Visual Impairment and Blindness*. 1981;2:41-45.

Stotland J. Relationship of parents to professionals: a challenge to professionals. *The Journal of Visual Impairment and Blindness*. 1984;2:69-74.

Chapter 10

Case Histories

- Be careful not to "pigeonhole" your patients into particular groups. Each patient, even among those with the same diagnosis, will have unique individual needs. The low vision provider's challenge is to *understand* each of these needs and offer as much assistance and support as possible.

- Patients needs can be met in the low vision clinic or through referral.

- Offer, but do not force suggestions on patients who are resistant to them. Remember that success or failure depends largely on an individual's personality.

The various parts of a low vision examination have been covered in previous chapters of this book. Each part of the examination and referral procedure was treated separately. In actual practice, however, the examination is a cohesive unit, not the sum of individual unrelated tests. The following cases are presented to illustrate how several extensive low vision evaluations might flow. Each patient represents someone who has been seen in low vision clinics and rehabilitation centers. Following these patients along through their low vision visit should help you get a feel for how to approach the individuals who will come for low vision care. In reading the case histories, remember that the suggestions given are just that. They are only suggestions. For each patient, there may be many right answers. Whatever choice is made, if the individual is able to accomplish his or her goals, the low vision visit has been a success.

The case histories represent extensive or unusual low vision cases. Try to remember, however, that low vision care is a part of a "normal" patient examination as well. Use the techniques for acuity testing for any patient whose vision falls below the 20/80 level, even temporarily. You will always have a more accurate assessment of vision. Use the techniques for determining increased power of reading glasses for any patient with a need for bifocal power greater than +3.00 diopters (D). Use the information on psychology of visual loss for all patients, even those who are simply postoperative cataract patients. These techniques can and should be used routinely. When low vision care becomes a part of normal patient management, the extra help needed by the more severely impaired patients will be second nature. Only then will we be providing optimum care to all patients.

Case One: Delores J.

Delores is a 72-year-old woman with bilateral intraocular lenses and macular degeneration in both eyes. She has had macular laser treatment in the left eye. Delores has been only a moderate reader all her life. She enjoys magazines and the daily newspaper. She also reads recipes and her mail. Since her vision has deteriorated she misses reading and writing letters and reading the daily newspaper. She has particular problems seeing the fine print of the obituaries and her Bible.

Delores came to the exam alone via a senior bus. She is a widow who lives alone in a retirement center where she takes her meals in a common dining room. A maid, provided by the center, comes once a week to vacuum, dust, change the bed linens, and clean the bathroom. During the exam Delores talks mainly about missing her family and being alone. She adjusts well to near reading distances, but becomes distracted easily. It is difficult to decide if she will remember much of what you tell her. General frailty and weakness causes her to have a slight hand tremor.

Exam:

Current prescription (Rx) and acuity level:

Right eye (OD): +1.00 -2.75 × 170 add +3.00 (acuity 10/80) (20/160 equivalent)

Left eye (OS): +1.75 -2.00 × 006 add +3.00 (acuity 10/400) (20/800 equivalent)

Near acuity with current Rx: 3M+ with both eyes (OU) together at 33 cm.

Low vision refractometric measurement (done in trial frame):

OD: +0.75 -2.00 × 170 (acuity 10/70)

OS: +1.75 -3.25 × 005 (acuity 10/400)

Near evaluation at 40 cm with +2.50 adds (over low vision refraction results):

OD: 3M+ (so near acuity is 40/3M or 40 cm/300 cm)

OS: The reading ability is so poor that it will not be a consideration when deciding lens power.

Trials with low vision aids:
- From the near acuity, 300 ÷ 40 = 7.50 so, a +7.50 reading add is tried for OD at near. Adding this to the distance correction, the total near prescription would be: +8.25 - 2.00 × 165.
- With the near Rx in a trial frame—She is able to read 1.5M print, 1M if the paper is steadied.
- With a +8.00 hand magnifier—She is unable to use the hand magnifier because of arm weakness. The magnifier shakes, and the focal distance is difficult to control.
- With a +9.00 stand magnifier and her current bifocal—She can read 1M, but has difficulty holding the magnifier in the correct position. It slides down the page and she loses her place easily.

Suggested Recommendations:
1. Reading spectacles as follows:
   OD: +8.25 -2.00 × 165 (This is the result of low vision refractometry with +7.50 add.) In the other eye, a balance prescription is adequate. Because of the poor vision OS, no base-in prism will be necessary in the reading glasses. She will read monocularly. If the vision from the poorer seeing eye interferes with her ability to read, that lens can be occluded or fogged.
2. Suggest a reading stand to hold the material still and maintain a constant reading distance. This is especially important because she has a hand tremor.
3. Suggest a reading lamp with a 60-watt bulb, reflective shade, and moveable arm. Experiment with the patient to decide what placement of the light provides her optimum illumination of reading material without glare.
4. Advise the use of a black felt-tip marker for writing letters. Suggest that she ask her family members to use one in correspondence to her as well.
5. Teach her to use a typoscope-style template for addressing envelopes.
6. Try a 4.7 D stand paperweight magnifier for use with her low vision spectacles for reading obituaries, phone book listings, and other small print. Usually, if someone can read 1.5 M with glasses, this magnifier is just enough to allow reading of 1M print (Figure 10-1). This stand magnifier is heavy, so it will not slide around easily if bumped. However, it will easily slide down a slanted reading stand. Instruct Delores to use it only on a flat surface.
7. Recommend a large-print or recorded Bible and give her addresses of where to acquire them.
8. Refer her to a rehabilitation teacher for a home visit. This will be to assist in organizing cabinets, marking dials on her stove, and the like. It will not be complicated, as most of her tasks of daily living are already taken care of by the staff at her residential center.
9. Order the aids and reading stand through your office, or provide them from your stock. She would find it difficult to order them herself, and with the lack of family support the aids would likely remain unordered.
10. Contact the retirement center to see if a social worker is on staff. This person should coordinate someone (family member, friend, staff member, or volunteer) who can also be taught the proper use of the spectacles, magnifier, and nonoptical aids. This way

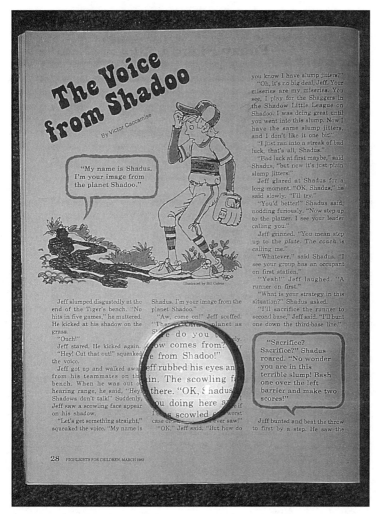

Figure 10-1. A paper-weight magnifier enlarges regular print approximately 2×, or to the size of large type.

Delores will have support in her home setting to ensure greater success.

11. Through the same social worker or a social service agency, recommend a community support group or visiting friends organization to offer her companionship. Her house of worship is another place to look for support, especially because reading the Bible seems to be important to her.

12. Have her return *with* her helper for follow-up in 2 to 3 weeks. You may need more than one follow-up visit because she is easily distracted. In her loneliness, she may not be motivated to try the aids right away.

Case Two: Harry E.

Harry is a 46-year-old man with proliferative diabetic retinopathy who has undergone panretinal photocoagulation multiple times in each eye. His insulin only keeps his blood sugar in fair control. He has difficulty walking as a result of diabetic-related neuropathy, and has relinquished his job as an electrician as a result of the visual and physical disabilities. He would like to work if medically possible. He can no longer drive because his vision is below legal limits. He is very photophobic and wears sunglasses even indoors.

He lives with his wife who does the cooking, cleaning, and driving. He enjoys lifting weights for exercise and has an extensive coin collection. Emotionally, he seems very motivated to try new magnifiers or anything that will help him with his work and daily life. His vision has been poor for quite a while and he is well-adjusted to his disability with realistic expectations and a good support network. He is impatient to get started with low vision services and regain some independence.

Exam:

Current Rx and acuity level:

OD: +1.25 -0.50 × 072 (acuity 20/70)

OS: +0.75 -0.75 × 105 (acuity 20/50-) He is able to see letters only in certain areas. He reads slowly.

Near acuity with current Rx: 2.5M with OU together, at a normal reading distance. There is no bifocal in the glasses.

Low vision refractometric measurement: (in the refractor)

OD: +1.00 -0.75 × 075 (acuity 20/70+)

OS: +1.00 -0.75 × 105 (acuity 20/50-)

Near evaluation at 40 cm with +2.50 adds (over low vision refractometry results):

OU: 1.5M print can be read (So near acuity is 40/1.5M or 40 cm/150 cm.)

Trials with low vision aids:

- From the near acuity 150 ÷ 40 = 3.75, so start with a +3.75 reading add.
- With +3.75 add—He reads 1M, but with hesitation. He misses some letters and words, so he has to struggle a bit to put sentences together. It is not the clarity of individual letters that seem to be a problem; rather, there are irregular "holes" in his field of view.
- +4.00 reading adds offer no improvement.

Suggested Recommendations:

1. The use of regular bifocals as follows:

   OD: +1.00 -0.75 × 075 add 3.75

   OS: +1.00 -0.75 × 105 add 3.75

   Make him aware that there are areas of his retina with scotomas, so the print may come and go in certain spots. He should practice using preferred areas of his retina, which may take some training and practice in the office. Larger print or higher magnification may make the problem more pronounced, as fewer letters will fit onto the healthy retinal areas.

2. Try bifocal lenses with a light absorbing tint for help with the photophobia. Check with your local optician or the New York Lighthouse for specifics. Absorptive sunglasses should be prescribed for outdoor use.

3. Practice with lighting for reading. Because glare is a problem, Harry may need less light from an indirect angle. A diffuser or filter over the shade may help. The absorptive filters in spectacles mentioned above may also be used while reading and writing. Yellow sunglasses or filters increase contrast of the printed page and may be used in lower light situations with good effect.

4. Try a 12 D illuminated stand magnifier for looking at his coin collection. The internal illumination will decrease glare, and the high power will be necessary to see the minute dates and markings.

5. Although he is able to read with standard reading adds, he may find other types of aids more to his advantage. Because he is motivated, he may be a good candidate for a closed circuit television (CCTV). It could help him even in his work. Perhaps he could find an electrician-related job doing planning or electrical engineering if he is able to see the appropriate plans and texts with the help of a CCTV.

6. Refer Harry to your state visual rehabilitation agency for complete vocational evaluation and training. This training should be based on the recommendation of his primary care physician. He will be eligible for many services based on his age and employability as long as his medical disability does not interfere with his ability to work. The vocational counsellor will probably recommend that the state help pay for aids and appliances, and may cover the cost of the CCTV and any retraining necessary to guarantee employment. He may have some difficulty being accepted for services based solely on his acuity level, as it is not within the category of legal blindness. However, because of his other disabilities, his young age, and his motivation, he will most likely be accepted.

7. Provide a catalogue of nonoptical low vision aids for his personal use. You might specifically suggest large-print watches and calculators.

8. Schedule a 2 week follow-up visit to evaluate the appropriateness of the spectacles and sunglasses for his daily needs.

Case Three: Claire I.

Claire is a 6-year-old girl with ocular albinism who came to the low vision clinic with her parents by referral from the school where she attends first grade. The parents feel that she does not need any help because she is functioning as well as a sighted child. She can run and play with other children, see small details, and is progressing in reading. The school recommendations are unclear and no teacher is present at the exam.

Exam:
Current Rx and acuity level:
OD: no correction (acuity 10/100)
OS: no correction (acuity 10/120)
Near acuity: 1M easily at close range without correction. She holds reading material at a distance of about 4 inches.

Low vision refractometry: (in trial frame without cycloplegia) (If the evaluation is difficult, it should be repeated with cycloplegia.)
OD: -0.50 sphere (acuity 10/100)
OS: -0.75 -0.50 × 075 (acuity 10/120)
Near: Acuity at 40 cm distance. Reads 3M. Near acuity is 40/3M.
Distance: With a trial of a 6× monocular telescope she can read 20/20 with either eye.

Suggested recommendations:
1. The power needed for reading at near is 300 ÷ 40, or +7.50 D. It is not necessary to provide any near low vision aid. They would only be cumbersome and are not needed because this 6-year-old girl has sufficient accommodation to focus the +7.50 without fatigue. Mention to Claire and her parents that she will eventually need

magnification at near as her accommodative ability diminishes and print size of texts decreases. First graders usually read 18-point type in their books and workbooks.

2. Recommend a monocular handheld 6× telescope for distance use. Encourage its use at school for seeing the chalkboard or for any distance activity. Arrange for training in the use of the telescope.

3. Encourage Claire's parents to let her use the telescope. Discuss the way her needs may change in the future. Mention that using an aid at an early age helps acceptance and removes negative stigma that occur later in life when "forced" to accept it.

4. Contact the teacher about school needs. Explain the use of the telescope and obtain recommendations about distance visual needs. Invite the teacher to attend the next visit if possible.

5. Provide a list of agencies serving the needs of visually impaired children and support groups for families. Refer Claire to the state agency for the visually impaired for services.

6. Schedule a follow-up visit for 1 year to reassess the situation. Because Claire's parents are reluctant to admit that she needs intervention, they should be encouraged to make decisions annually about how to approach her changing visual and educational needs. Also, as her accommodative reserves decrease and her visual demands increase she will experience new needs and require changes to her recommended optical aids.

Follow-up note: in this actual situation, the parents declined the telescope and all other suggestions. They wanted to return for follow-up when they felt Claire needed some help. They did not want her to appear "different" or to be treated differently by other children.

Case Four: Doris M.

Doris is a 64-year-old woman with macular degeneration. She is very intelligent and an avid reader. In the past, she visited a low vision clinic where she was successfully prescribed an appropriate low vision aid. Now she complains that she can no longer see as well with her 12 D half-eye spectacles. She wants to be able to continue reading books for pleasure.

She is involved with many civic organizations and activities. Her husband drives and takes care of the family finances, they share the household duties. Cooking and cleaning are not a problem for her, but she cannot read price tags while shopping.

Exam:

Current Rx and acuity level:

OD: no correction (10/120)

OS: no correction (10/160)

During acuity testing she states that she can see the small title on the test better than those huge numbers. This seems peculiar, but an attempt is made to recheck the acuity with smaller optotypes. Sometimes there is a minimal area of intact retina that will only allow resolution of an image within its small area.

Acuity test using smaller characters:

OD: 10/20, one letter at a time (This is a 20/40 equivalent.)

OS: 10/160

Near acuity with current +12 spectacles: OD: 2M, OS: 3M (eccentrically).

Low vision refractometry (in trial frame):

OD: -2.00 -0.75 × 163 (10/20+)

OS: -2.25 -1.25 × 075 (10/160)

Near evaluation at 40 cm with +2.50 adds: reads 1M print (with OD only), so acuity is 40/1M.

- Trial with +5.00 adds: 2M-

The visual field assessment is especially important in this patient to determine the number and size of the areas of useful vision in the macular area.

Tangent screen: Intact peripheral fields in both eyes. Central scotomas OU.

Amsler grid: Central scotomas OU, but a small parafoveal area remains clear OD.

Suggested recommendations:

1. Doris prefers to read with her small island of intact macula. When images are magnified, they are too large to be seen within the limits of her small usable field of macular vision. As larger images must be viewed with peripheral retina, her vision actually diminishes with magnification. Because her low vision refractometric measurement has a -2.50 spherical equivalent, a +2.50 add renders her near prescription essentially plano and she can read without correction. If she notes a subjective improvement from the cylinder correction, reading glasses can be suggested.

2. Encourage her to read using her area of excellent vision. Advise her that the vision she has will not be destroyed by use. She had noticed she could see some things without her glasses, but was afraid to try, thinking it would hurt her eyes. If her eyes become fatigued, she can use her +12.00 spectacles or return for a stronger Rx.

3. Recommend a reading lamp for indoors and a penlight for reading price tags in stores.

4. A catalogue of nonoptical aids should be provided to help her with her daily activities. Even though she states that everything is fine, she will find some aids and appliances that will ease her work.

5. Doris could help you set up a support group for patients with similar visual loss. With her energy and interest in civic organizations she will be a valuable volunteer in reaching out to other patients.

6. Provide information on where to acquire large print reading materials.

Case Five: Michael D.

Michael is an 83-year-old man with glaucoma and macular degeneration. His left eye has no light perception from a central retinal vein occlusion and neovascular glaucoma. One year ago he underwent cataract extraction with intraocular lens (IOL) in the right eye, but suffered some complications including elevated intraocular pressure. His vision has remained stable for 6 months. Michael is unable to read his own mail or balance his checkbook. He misses reading very much. His wife does all the household chores. He is very discouraged and poorly motivated. He thinks nothing will help him and that his productive life has ended.

Exam:

Current Rx and acuity level:

OD: -1.00 -1.75 × 100 add 2.25 (acuity 20/80)

OS: balance Rx with no light perception

Near acuity with current Rx: 2M with difficulty.

Low vision refractometry:

OD: -1.50 -1.50 × 105 (20/60)

Near evaluation at 40 cm with +2.50 add: reads 2M more easily (acuity is 40/2M)

- 200 ÷ 40 = 5.00, so try a +5.00 add—able to read 1M print.
- With actual reading material he is able to read a checkbook and newspaper, but complains about the vision and shows poor motivation to try aids at home.

Suggested recommendations:

1. Patients like Michael are very difficult. Their discouragement may result in rejecting everything you tell them. Or they may get home and be more motivated than other patients who are excited about their visual improvement when in your office. In the face of success, Michael is still complaining he cannot see.
2. Provide him with 6 D half-eye spectacles and a 5 D hand magnifier to take home on the condition he promises to try them and come back to report about his successes and failures in 2 weeks. This will allow him to try the aids in his home environment, and ensure that he returns for follow-up so you can have at least one more try.

Follow-up with Michael D.:

In 2 weeks he returned for follow-up and rejected the spectacles completely. He had no interest in the close reading distance. He said the magnifier was okay but it did not make the print quite as dark as he would like it. A trial with a 6 D aspheric magnifier proved more successful.

New suggestions:

1. Provide the 6-D magnifier.
2. Reiterate and train Michael and his wife on the importance of magnifier-to-page distance appropriate to a 6-D lens (16.6 cm).
3. Discuss proper lighting and recommend a reading lamp.
4. Suggest a pocket magnifier for use outside the home.
5. Give a lot of reassurance and recommend some social service agencies and support groups, particularly if he has not yet been referred to the state agency for the blind.
6. Schedule another follow-up visit in 3 months in case he is ready to accept more aids, and to ensure that the current ones are being used correctly. Michael will need continual reassurance. Be sure he leaves your office with a stack of reference material, a nonoptical aids catalogue, and a large print calling card. Someday he may decide he wants help. He then can refer to these materials.

Case Six: Susan M.

Susan is a 34-year-old woman with congenital nystagmus and high myopia. She has had poor vision all her life, but has always been able to read without glasses because of the magnification provided by uncorrected high myopia. She had retinal detachment surgery in her right eye at age 17, and strabismus surgery for exotropia at age 7. Two years ago she developed cataracts during pregnancy and her vision decreased dramatically. She had cataract extraction with IOL OD 2 months ago. The cataract remains in the left eye, but does not limit the vision quite as much.

Susan leads a very active life and has a husband and two children. She wants to be able to read again, and to play Mah-Jongg with her friends. She is vibrant and extremely motivated to try anything you can offer. Although she has had no low vision help in the past, she is well-adjusted to her disability and has very specific needs. (This is the ideal patient.)

Exam:

Current Rx and acuity level:

OD: no glasses since surgery (acuity 10/300)

OS: -6.00 -3.00 × 180 (acuity 10/120)

Near acuity with current Rx: 5M with glasses on, 1.5M with glasses off because of the high myopia OS, but only when held at a very close distance. It is "foggy" because of the cataract.

Low vision refractometry:

OD: +4.50 -2.00 × 180 (10/40)

OS: -7.50 -2.75 × 180 (10/100)

Near acuity with +2.50 adds at 40 cm: 1.5M (acuity is 40/1.5M)

- 150 ÷ 40 = 3.75, so try +3.75 add—She reads 1M, but with difficulty.
- With +5.00 adds—She reads 1M very easily, can read Mah-Jongg rules, and is *thrilled* with the vision.

Suggested Recommendations:

1. The major issue in this case is the anisometropia, or huge difference between the refractive powers of the two eyes. Most patients would not tolerate this prescription because of the difference in image size when viewed with either eye. The glasses would also be cosmetically unusual because the lenses would look very different from one another. In Susan's case, she is not bothered by the image size difference because she alternately suppresses each eye. To balance the look of the glasses her left eye could be given a balance lens of +4.00. This would overcorrect the left eye by 11.5 D and offer magnification for near viewing as well. Because she likes to alternate fixation, however, the 11.5 D overcorrection creates an annoying blur when trying to view with the left eye. The correct glasses prescription was actually preferred by Susan although it is very unusual. Another way to overcome the cosmesis problem is to correct one eye with a contact lens so the overcorrection can be balanced. Sometimes, if the second eye comes to cataract surgery the intraocular lens power is adjusted to more closely balance the two eyes. Unfortunately, this is not always an ideal answer. In Susan's case, she relies on her myopic left eye to provide magnification for reading without glasses. If after cataract surgery she was made hyperopic in that eye to balance with the other, she would lose her functional reading ability OS.

2. Her glasses should have a +3.00 bifocal add for near viewing. This will allow normal viewing, card playing, and Mah-Jongg playing at table distance.

3. A separate pair of reading glasses with the increased +5.00 add power will allow actual reading of smaller print.

4. Provide a 10 D hand magnifier for shopping so she does not have to keep changing glasses.

5. Discuss lighting. She may be light sensitive and desire a pair of absorptive filter sunglasses.

6. Work with telescopes for distant objects. She would require only a very low power, but it could be helpful for things like watching her child's ballet recital or school play.

7. She may be a good candidate for a CCTV if she wants to work, go to school, etc. Mention the existence of these machines, and arrange a trial with one in her home if she is interested.

8. Refer her to the state agency for the blind so she can get any services she may need. She may benefit from vocational counselling or the services of a rehabilitation teacher.

A Glossary of Basic Optical Terms

This book presumes that the reader has a basic understanding of optics and optical principles. Because some low vision assistants are new to the field, they may not have the background to fully understand some of the information. This is a *brief* description of optical principles in dictionary form to help with the comprehension of these topics. For a more thorough discussion of optics, refer to the following texts:

Rubin M. *Optics for Clinicians*. Gainesville, Fl: TRIAD Scientific Publishers; 1974.

Bryant M. *Optics, Retinoscopy and Refractometry*. Thorofare, NJ: SLACK Incorporated; 1997. In press.

Accommodation

Accommodation is the natural ability of the physiologic lens to make itself thicker or thinner in response to image distance, in order to allow that image to be focused on the retina. Closer image distances require higher powers of accommodation. The natural aging process causes accommodative ability to diminish, a process referred to as presbyopia.

Convergence

Convergence of light rays occurs when the more peripheral rays in a bundle bend inward toward the central ray or optical axis. Convergence is measured in plus diopters. Convergence does not occur "naturally." Light rays only converge after passing through a plus lens. Convergence is also the term used to describe the turning inward of both eyes to focus on a near object.

Diopter

A diopter (D) is the unit of measurement for lenses. One diopter is the power of a lens that will focus parallel rays of light at a distance of 1 m.

Divergence

Divergence of light rays occurs when the more peripheral rays in a bundle bend outward away from the central ray or optical axis. Divergence is measured in minus diopters. Divergence is the natural vergence that occurs as light travels through space.

Focal Distance

Focal distance is the distance at which converging light rays come to a point of focus behind a plus lens. If the rays striking the front of a lens are parallel, the focal distance is determined by the formula $F=1/D$, where F is the focal length, 1 is one meter (or 100 cm), and D is the dioptric power of the lens. To determine the focal distance of a lens, divide 100 cm by the power of the lens. The result is the focal distance in centimeters.

Lens

A lens is a curved piece of glass, plastic, or other transparent material. When light rays pass through a spherical lens, the central ray passes through undeviated. Peripheral light rays are refracted, or caused to diverge or converge in relation to the central ray.

Light Rays

When light leaves its source it travels in rays. These are individual "pencils" of light that continue to travel forward undeviated in their course until affected by a lens or other refractive material. The rays travel in bundles that diverge in relation to one another.

Magnification

This refers to the enlargement in the size of an image. Magnification is measured in dioptric power or in terms of ×. (This book refers to magnification in diopters.)

Motion Parallax

Telescopes and other magnifiers have reduced fields of view. As an image is viewed through the small visual aperture, objects pass through the small field very quickly. This apparent motion is much faster than normal. If the telescope itself is moved, the apparent motion is also much faster. This apparent motion is known as motion parallax.

Optical Axis

The optical axis is the central ray of a bundle of light rays that passes through the exact center of a lens. There is no divergence or convergence. It is the ray of optimal and constant focus.

Optical Infinity

Optical infinity is the distance at which bundles of light rays no longer have any measurable divergence. The light rays are referred to as being parallel, or as having "zero vergence." In reality light rays never stop diverging, but the divergence becomes too small to detect at optical infinity. In clinical optics, infinity is presumed to occur at 20 ft (or 6 m). In geometric optics, infinity is less clearly understood and occurs at "infinity," however you choose to define it.

Prism

A prism is a lens, but is not curved. The front and back surfaces of a prism are both flat, and are arranged at an angle to each other so there is a thick end (the base) and a thin end (the apex). Prisms cause bundles of light rays to bend in one direction instead of toward or away from the optical center. As a result, images are not focused, but are shifted in the direction of the apex of the prism. One prism diopter moves images 1 cm toward the apex of the prism at a focal distance of 1 m. Larger displacements can be achieved by increasing the power of the prism or increasing the distance from which the object is viewed.

Refraction

Refraction is the bending of light rays by a lens. Convex (plus) lenses cause light rays to converge. Concave (minus) lenses cause light rays to diverge.

Scanning

Scanning refers to the technique of looking across a particular area by sweeping a magnifier or telescope slowly in a horizontal fashion to take in the complete field of view. It requires moving the lens, so motion parallax may interfere.

Spotting

Spotting is the technique of finding and viewing a stationary object in the field of view. Neither the eye nor the lens are moved.

Tracking

Tracking is the technique of viewing a moving object. The object and the magnifier are both in motion, so keeping them aligned can be tricky. Motion parallax and smearing of the view are common problems, as is losing the view of the object altogether.

Vergence

Vergence is the moving apart or together of light rays in a bundle. In regard to lenses, there are two vergences. First is the vergence of the rays before they strike the lens, which is dependent on distance travelled from the source. Second is the resultant vergence as the light rays leave the lens after having been refracted. The formula to determine this is $U+P=V$ where U is the unaffected vergence of the light rays just as they strike the front surface of the lens, P is the power of the lens, and V is the resultant vergence of the rays just as they leave the back surface of the lens. Vergence is measured in diopters.

Virtual Image

A virtual image appears optically to be somewhere other than its actual location.

Internet Addresses of Low Vision Resources

Web Pages With Links to Multiple Agencies and Associations Related to Blind and Low Vision Topics

Blindness-Related Resources on the Web and Beyond: (exhaustive list and links with frequent updates) http://www.hicom.net/~oedipus/blind.html

Scotter's Low Vision Land: (Entertaining and informative webpage with multiple links) http://www.community.net:80/~byndsght

Specific Vendors Mentioned in This Book

Blazie Engineering: http://www.blazie.com

HumanWare, Inc: http://www.humanware.com

LS&S Group, Inc: http://www.lssgroup.com

Telesensory Corp: http://www.telesensory.com

Specific Agencies Mentioned in This Book

The American Council of the Blind: http://www.acb.org

American Foundation for the Blind: gopher://gopher.afb.org:5005/

American Printing House for the Blind: http://www.aph.org

National Federation of the Blind: http://www.nfb.org

National Library Service for the Blind and Physically Handicapped: http://lcweb.loc.gov/ nls/nls.html

Other Agencies of Interest

ADA Information Center On-line: http://www.idir.net/~adabbs/rblind.html

Blind Children's Center: http://www.blindcntr.org/bcc

Center for Independent Living: http://www.wenet.net/~cil

Digital Journal of Ophthalmology: http://www.meei.harvard.edu/meei/DJOhome.html

Guiding Eyes for the Blind: http://www.guiding-eyes.org

National Society to Prevent Blindness: http://www.carnscape.com/preblind.html

The On-line Books Page: http://www.cs.cmu.edu/web/books.html

Special Needs Education Network: http://sne.ingenia.com

Index

ACB. *See* American Council of the Blind

acceptance of vision loss, determination of, 49-50

accommodation, 71, 125

acuity, versus lens power, 71

Agencies and support groups, 74, 79-81, 94, 115, 118, 131

American Council of the Blind (ACB), 80, 131

American Diabetes Association, 81, 131

American Foundation for the Blind (AFB), 42, 80-81, 131

American Printing House for the Blind, 34, 37, 42, 131

Amsler grid test, 64

appliances, household, adapted to low vision patients, 36

assistant, low vision, role of, 5

Association for Education and Rehabilitation of the Blind and Visually Impaired, 81

Astigmatism, detection of, 60-61

bioptics, 23-24

Blind Children's Center, 131

Blindness: What It Is, What It Does, and How to Live With It (Carroll), 99-102

Braille, 37-38, 81-82

computer adaptations of, 40

National Braille Press, 37

canes, white, 83

career, loss of, after vision loss, 100

Carroll, Thomas J, 99

Center for Independent Living, 131

children, patient history, 52-54

clinic, low vision, 4, 89-95

equipment for, 91-93

referrals to, 94-95, 105

community involvement of clinic, 95

compression of speech, 41-42

computer-assisted reading and writing technology, 35, 38-42

computer programs for low vision users, 39, 40

convergence, definition of, 125

Council of Citizens with Low Vision, 80

counselors, rehabilitation, 82

diabetes mellitus, 32, 38, 47, 59, 113-115

diagnosis codes, for low vision services, 95

Digital Journal of Ophthalmology, 131

diopters, 10, 12, 125

diopter/distance chart, 11

and focal distance, 72

magnification power equivalencies, 12

and M unit equivalents, 70-71

Directory of Agencies Serving the Blind and Visually Handicapped in the US, 81

distance acuity testing, 59-60

divergence, definition of, 125

dogs, guide, 83

driving, 23-24, 47

education institutions for low-vision patients, 87

education of patients, 51-52

family and friends, problems with, 102

financial concerns, 74-75

financial security, loss of, after vision loss, 101

Focal distance

definition of, 125

and dioptric power, 72

focal length, 10-12

follow-up visits, 73-74

games adapted to low vision patients, 36-37

Guiding Eyes for the Blind, 131

Hadley School for the Blind, 79

Helen Keller National Center for Deaf-Blind Youth and Adults, 81

help for patients

agencies and support groups, 74, 79-81, 94, 115-118, 131

financial, 74-75

rehabilitation personnel, 82-87

hobbies adapted to low vision patients, 36-37

HOTV distance test chart, 92, 93

HOTV near card, 92

household appliances adapted to low vision patients, 36

Internet addresses, 131

large print, 33-35, 40-41

legal blindness, 104

definition of, 3-4

lens, definition of, 125

lens power, versus acuity, 71

Lighthouse, Inc, 80-81

lighting, 31-33

light rays, definition of, 125

Lions Club, and financial help, 74-75

loupes, 21-22
low vision aids, sources for, 27, 131
low vision care, history of, 3
Low Vision Chart Set, 91
low vision, definition of, 3
Low Vision Starter Kit® (Jose), 91

magnification, 9, 125
    power equivalencies, 12
    for specific patients, 70-72
magnifiers
    hand, 15-18
    stand, 18-21
medical devices adapted to low vision patients, 36
Medicare, 74
microscopes, 14
motion parallax, 23, 125
M units, 62
    and dioptric equivalents, 70-71
myopic patients, 71

NAPVI. *See* National Association for Parents of
    the Visually Impaired
National Association for Parents of the Visually
    Impaired (NAPVI), 79-80, 106
National Association for the Visually Handicapped
    (NAVH), 33-34, 80
National Federation of the Blind, 80, 131
National Library Service for the Blind and Physi-
    cally Handicapped (NLS), 33-34, 42, 81, 131
National Society to Prevent Blindness, 131
NAVH. *See* National Association for the Visually
    Handicapped
Near vision testing, 62-63
New York Times Large Type Weekly, 34
NLS. *See* National Library Service for the Blind
    and Physically Handicapped
Nonoptical aids, 31-48, 91
    sources of, 42

occupational therapists, 87
On-Line Books Page, 131
optical aids, 12-26, 91
optical axis, definition of, 126
optical infinity, definition of, 126
orientation and mobility (O&M) instructors, 82-87
patient(s)
    acceptance of vision loss, determining, 49-50
    age of, and accommodative ability, 71
    educating, 51-52, 72-74

emotional care of, 4, 47-49, 51-52, 59, 99-106
input to aid selection, 72-74
support for
    by family and friends, determining level
        of, 50-51
    sources for, 79-81
    training of, 73-74, 82-87
vision needs of, determining, 47-49
winning trust of, 51-52

patient history, 47, 52-54, 69-70
    form for, 55
peripatologists, 82-87
practitioners, functions of, 4
pricing, for low vision services, 95
prism, definition of, 126
public schools, and cost deferral, 74

rapport with patient, 51-52
Reader's Digest Large Type Edition, 34
reading aids, 33-35
referral agencies, 94
referrals, to low vision clinics, 94-95, 105
refraction, definition of, 126
refractive error, 12
    and choosing lens power, 71-72
    verification of, 60-61
rehabilitation personnel, 82-87
Retinitis Pigmentosa Foundation, 81

safety glasses, 53
scanning, definition of, 126
self-image, changes in, after vision loss, 99-102
set-up, of low vision service, 89-95
sighted guide training, 84-87
social service agencies, 74, 79, 94, 115, 118
    referrals to, 5, 52
Special Needs Education Network, 131
spectacles, 12-15, 13
speech compression, 41-42
speech, synthesized, 39-41
sports associations for low-vision patients, 81
spotting, definition of, 126
state agencies, 79, 94, 115, 118
sunglasses, 32-33, 91
support groups and agencies, 74, 79-81, 94, 115,
    118, 131
support groups, creation of, 105
support of family and friends, determining level
    of, 50-51

synthesized speech machines, 39-41

teachers, rehabilitation, 82
telemicroscopes, 14, 24-26
telescopes, 22-26
    bioptic, 23-24
    handheld, 22-23, 25, 26
television, closed circuit, as reading aid, 38-39
tracking, 26, 126
training, for low vision patients, 73-74, 82-87
trials, of low-vision aid
    at home, 73
    in office, 72-73
trust of patient, winning, 51-52
typoscopes, 69

vendors, for low vision products, 27, 40-42, 131
vergence, definition of, 126
Veterans Administration, and cost deferral, 74
virtual image, definition of, 126
vision aids
    choosing for specific patient, 69-75

and financial concerns, 74-75
nonoptical, 31-48
optical, 12-26, 91
for reading, 33-35
selection of, step-by-step guide, 75
sources for, 27, 40-42, 131
for writing, 33-35
vision assessment
    distance acuity, 59-60
    near vision, 62-63, 70
    refractive error, 60-61
vision assessment, step-by-step guide, 65
Vision Resource List, 81
visual efficiency, definition of, 3
visual field loss, 63-64
Visually Impaired Information Specialists, Inc, 81

web pages, for low vision topics, 131
writing aids, 33-35

Xerox Imaging System, 40
X notation, 11, 12

For your information

This book and many others on numerous different topics are available from SLACK Incorporated. For further information or a copy of our latest catalog, contact us at:

Professional Book Division
SLACK Incorporated
6900 Grove Road
Thorofare, NJ 08086 USA
Telephone: 1-609-848-1000
1-800-257-8290
Fax: 1-609-853-5991
E-mail: orders@slackinc.com
WWW: http://www.slackinc.com

We accept most major credit cards and checks or money orders in US dollars drawn on a US bank. Most orders are shipped within 72 hours.

Contact us for information on recent releases, forthcoming titles, and bestsellers. If you have a comment about this title or see a need for a new book, direct your correspondence to the Editorial Director at the above address.

*If you are an instructor, we can be reached at the address listed above or on the Internet at **educomps@slackinc.com** for specific needs.*

Thank you for your interest and we hope you found this work beneficial.